PCOS COOKBOOK FOR WOMEN

The Complete Guide With
Delicious Recipes To Manage
And Balance your Hormones
And Improve Fertility

Derek Klein

TABLE OF CONTENTS

Introduction

I still remember the day I received my PCOS diagnosis. It felt like a punch in the gut - a mix of emotions that left me feeling lost and alone. But as I began to navigate this new reality, I realized that I wasn't alone. Millions of women worldwide were facing the same struggles, the same frustrations, and the same fears.

As I delved deeper into understanding PCOS, I discovered that food could be a powerful tool in managing my symptoms. But it wasn't just about cutting out certain foods or following a specific diet - it was about nourishing my body with whole, nutritious foods that made me feel good, both physically and emotionally.

I started experimenting with new ingredients, cooking techniques, and flavor combinations. I devoured cookbooks, scoured the internet, and talked to other women with PCOS. And slowly but surely, I started to feel like I was taking control of my health.

The journey wasn't easy, though. There were setbacks, failures, and moments of frustration. But with each success, no matter how small, I felt a sense of empowerment that I had never felt before. I realized that I didn't have to be a slave to my symptoms, that I could rise above them and thrive.

That's when I started creating recipes that catered to my PCOS needs. I crafted dishes that balanced my blood sugar, boosted my mood, and nourished my body. I created meals that made me feel like I was living with PCOS, not suffering from it.

This cookbook is a culmination of that journey. It's a collection of recipes that have helped me thrive, despite PCOS. Recipes that have made me feel like I'm in control, like I'm living my best life. And I hope they will do the same for you.

In the following pages, you'll find over 80 recipes that are designed to nourish your body and soul. Recipes that are easy to make, delicious, and adaptable to your lifestyle. Recipes that will make you feel like you're taking control of your health, one delicious meal at a time.

Chapter One

Overview Of PCOS And Its Impact On Women's Health

Polycystic Ovary Syndrome (PCOS) is a hormonal disorder that affects women of reproductive age. It is a complex condition that impacts various aspects of women's health, including:

1. Reproductive System: PCOS is characterized by irregular menstrual cycles, cysts on the ovaries, and insulin resistance, leading to difficulties with ovulation and fertility.

2. Hormonal Imbalance: PCOS is marked by high levels of androgens (male hormones) and irregular estrogen levels, causing a range of symptoms.

3. Metabolic Health: Insulin resistance and metabolic dysfunction increase the risk of developing type 2 diabetes, cardiovascular disease, and weight-related issues.

4. Mental Health: Women with PCOS are more likely to experience depression, anxiety, and eating disorders due to the emotional impact of the condition.

5. Physical Health: PCOS is associated with various physical symptoms, including weight gain, acne, hair loss, and excessive hair growth.

6. Cardiovascular Health: Women with PCOS are at higher risk of developing high blood pressure, high cholesterol, and cardiovascular disease.

7. Sleep and Digestive Health: PCOS can lead to sleep apnea, insomnia, and digestive issues like bloating and constipation.

8. Bone Health: Women with PCOS may experience osteoporosis and osteopenia due to hormonal imbalances.

9. Autoimmune Disorders: PCOS is linked to an increased risk of autoimmune diseases like thyroiditis, rheumatoid arthritis, and lupus.

10. Quality of Life: PCOS can significantly impact a woman's overall well-being, self-esteem, and daily life, making it essential to seek medical attention and support.

It's important to note that every woman with PCOS may not experience all of these impacts, and the severity of the condition can vary widely. Early diagnosis, lifestyle changes, and medical treatment can help manage PCOS and improve overall health.

Importance Of Diet In Managing PCOS

Diet plays a crucial role in managing Polycystic Ovary Syndrome (PCOS). A well-planned diet can help alleviate symptoms, improve overall health, and increase fertility.

Importance of diet in managing PCOS:

1. Blood Sugar Control: PCOS is often associated with insulin resistance, which can lead to type 2 diabetes. A diet low in refined carbohydrates and added sugars helps regulate blood sugar levels.

2. Weight Management: Maintaining a healthy weight can improve insulin sensitivity, hormone balance, and fertility. A balanced diet with appropriate portion sizes and calorie intake supports weight management.

3. Hormone Regulation: Certain foods, such as phytoestrogens (e.g., soy, flaxseeds), can help regulate estrogen levels. Omega-3 fatty acids (e.g., salmon, walnuts) support hormone balance and reduce inflammation.

4. Inflammation Reduction: PCOS Is characterized by chronic inflammation. Antioxidant-rich foods (e.g., berries, leafy greens), omega-3 fatty acids, and turmeric help reduce inflammation.

5. Fertility Support: A diet rich in folic acid (e.g., dark leafy greens), iron (e.g., red meat, spinach), and omega-3 fatty acids supports fertility and prenatal health.

6. Digestive Health: PCOS is often linked to digestive issues like bloating and constipation. A diet high in fiber (e.g., whole grains, fruits), probiotics (e.g., yogurt, kefir), and healthy fats supports digestive health.

7. Micronutrient Adequacy: PCOS can increase the risk of micronutrient deficiencies (e.g., vitamin D, B12). A balanced diet ensures adequate intake of essential vitamins and minerals.

8. Reducing Androgen Levels: Foods like saw palmetto and spearmint tea may help reduce androgen levels, alleviating symptoms like acne and excessive hair growth.

9. Improving Mental Health: A healthy diet rich in omega-3 fatty acids, vitamin D, and magnesium supports mental health and reduces symptoms of depression and anxiety.

10. Overall Well-being: A balanced diet improves overall health, energy levels, and quality of life, enabling women with PCOS to better manage their condition.

By focusing on whole, nutrient-dense foods and avoiding processed and high-sugar foods, women with PCOS can take control of their diet and improve their overall health and well-being.

Goals And Objectives Of This Cookbook

The goals and objectives of this PCOS cookbook are:

1. Empower women with PCOS to take control of their diet and health

2. Provide delicious and nutritious recipes that cater to PCOS dietary needs

3. Help manage PCOS symptoms through balanced eating

4. Support weight management and improve insulin sensitivity

5. Regulate hormones and improve fertility

6. Reduce inflammation and improve overall health

7. Provide easy-to-follow recipes that fit into a busy lifestyle

8. Offer meal planning tips and grocery shopping guidance

9. Inspire holistic wellness and self-care practices

By achieving these goals, this cookbook aims to become a trusted resource and companion for women with PCOS, helping them navigate the journey towards better health and wellbeing.

Chapter Two

Understanding PCOS And Nutrition

Understanding PCOS and nutrition is crucial for managing the condition.
Key points to understand:

1. Balanced diet: Focus on whole, unprocessed foods like vegetables, fruits, whole grains, lean proteins, and healthy fats.

2. Carbohydrate management: Choose complex carbs with fiber, like whole grains and vegetables, to regulate blood sugar and insulin levels.

3. Protein and healthy fats: Include lean protein sources like poultry, fish, and legumes, and healthy fats like avocado, nuts, and olive oil.

4. Omega-3 rich foods: Include foods high in omega-3 fatty acids, like salmon, flaxseeds, and walnuts, to reduce inflammation.

5. Antioxidant-rich foods: Eat foods high in antioxidants, like berries, leafy greens, and other fruits and vegetables, to reduce oxidative stress.

6. Hydration: Drink plenty of water and limit sugary drinks.

7. Limit processed and high-sugar foods: Avoid foods that can exacerbate PCOS symptoms, like processed snacks, sugary drinks, and refined carbohydrates.

8. Individualized nutrition: Work with a healthcare provider or registered dietitian to develop a personalized nutrition plan that suits your specific needs.

By understanding the nutritional aspects of PCOS, you can make informed food choices to manage your symptoms, improve your overall health, and enhance your wellbeing.

What Is PCOS And How Does It Affect Metabolism And Hormones?

Polycystic Ovary Syndrome (PCOS) is a hormonal disorder that affects women of reproductive age. It is characterized by:

1. Irregular menstrual cycles: Infrequent or prolonged periods, or no periods at all.

2. Polycystic ovaries: Multiple small cysts on the ovaries, which can be detected by ultrasound.

3. Hormonal imbalance: High levels of androgens (male hormones) and irregular estrogen levels.

PCOS affects metabolism and hormones in several ways:

1. Insulin resistance: Many women with PCOS have insulin resistance, leading to high blood sugar levels and an increased risk of developing type 2 diabetes.

2. Androgen excess: High levels of androgens, such as testosterone, can cause acne, excessive hair growth, and male pattern baldness.

3. Estrogen imbalance: Irregular estrogen levels can lead to mood swings, fatigue, and weight gain.

4. Metabolic syndrome: PCOS is associated with an increased risk of metabolic syndrome, a cluster of conditions that increase the risk of developing type 2 diabetes and cardiovascular disease

5. Thyroid dysfunction: Some women with PCOS may experience thyroid dysfunction, particularly hypothyroidism (underactive thyroid)

6. Adrenal dysfunction: PCOS is also linked to adrenal dysfunction, leading to issues like cortisol imbalance and adrenal fatigue.

7. Hormonal imbalance: PCOS can disrupt the balance of other hormones, including prolactin, follicle-stimulating hormone (FSH), and luteinizing hormone (LH).

These hormonal and metabolic changes can lead to a range of symptoms, including weight gain, fatigue, mood swings, and infertility. Understanding the impact of PCOS on metabolism and hormones is crucial for developing effective treatment and management strategies.

The Role Of Nutrition In Managing PCOS Symptoms

Nutrition plays a crucial role in managing PCOS symptoms.
A well-planned diet can help:

1. Regulate blood sugar and insulin levels
2. Balance hormones
3. Reduce androgen levels
4. Improve menstrual regularity
5. Enhance fertility
6. Support weight management
7. Reduce inflammation
8. Improve mental health

Key nutritional strategies for managing PCOS symptoms include:

1. Balanced macronutrient intake
2. Whole, unprocessed foods
3. High fiber intake
4. Healthy fats and omega-3 fatty acids
5. Antioxidant-rich foods
6. Probiotics and gut health support
7. Adequate hydration
8. Limit processed and high-sugar foods

By focusing on nutrient-dense foods and a balanced diet, women with PCOS can better manage their symptoms and improve their overall health and wellbeing.

Key Nutrients And Supplements For PCOS Management

These are list of key nutrients and supplements that may help with PCOS management:

1. Omega-3 fatty acids: Reduce inflammation and improve hormone balance.

2. Vitamin D: Important for hormone regulation and insulin sensitivity.

3. Magnesium: Helps with insulin sensitivity, hormone balance, and menstrual regularity.

4. Chromium: Supports insulin sensitivity and blood sugar control.

5. Zinc: Essential for hormone regulation, immune function, and fertility.

6. B vitamins: Particularly B6, B9 (folate), and B12, which support hormone regulation and metabolism.

7. Antioxidants: Such as vitamin C, E, and beta-carotene, which help reduce oxidative stress and inflammation.

8. Probiotics: Support gut health, immune function, and hormone balance.

9. Inositol: Helps with insulin sensitivity, hormone balance, and menstrual regularity.

10. N-Acetyl Cysteine (NAC): Supports antioxidant defenses and hormone balance.

11. Vitamin K: Important for insulin sensitivity and bone health.

12. Coenzyme Q10 (CoQ10): Antioxidant that supports energy production and hormone balance.

13. Turmeric/Curcumin: Anti-inflammatory and antioxidant properties.

14. Ginseng: Supports insulin sensitivity and hormone balance.

15. Berberine: Supports insulin sensitivity and glucose metabolism.

Again, it's essential to consult with a healthcare provider before adding any supplements to your regimen, as they may interact with medications or have adverse effects in certain individuals. A balanced diet and lifestyle changes should always be the primary approach, with supplements used as additional support.

Chapter Three

Nourishing Breakfast Recipes

1. Berry Oatmeal Bowl

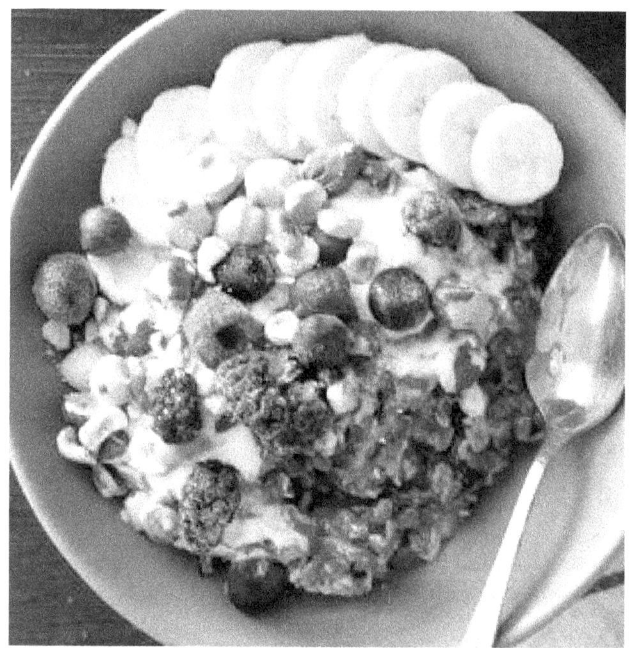

Ingredients:
- 1/2 cup rolled oats
- 1/2 cup unsweetened almond milk
- 1/4 cup mlxed berries (fresh or frozen)
- 1 tablespoon chia seeds

- 1 tablespoon honey or maple syrup (optional)
- 1/4 teaspoon ground cinnamon
- Pinch of salt
- Toppings (optional): sliced almonds, shredded coconut, Greek yogurt

Instructions:
1. In a pot, bring the almond milk to a simmer over medium heat.
2. Add the oats, chia seeds, honey or maple syrup (if using), cinnamon, and salt.
3. Reduce heat to low and cook, stirring occasionally, until the oats have absorbed most of the liquid and the mixture has a creamy consistency, about 5-7 minutes.
4. Stir in the mixed berries.
5. Pour into a bowl and add toppings (if using).
6. Serve warm and enjoy.

Tips:
- Use fresh or frozen mixed berries, such as blueberries, strawberries, and raspberries.
- Add a scoop of protein powder or nut butter for extra protein and creaminess.
- Substitute other non-dairy milk alternatives like soy milk or coconut milk if desired.
- Add a sprinkle of cinnamon or nutmeg for extra flavor.
- Make ahead: Cook the oats and chia seeds the night before and refrigerate, then top with berries and other toppings in the morning.

This recipe is PCOS-friendly because it includes:

- Whole grains (oats)
- Unsweetened almond milk (low in sugar and calories)
- Chia seeds (rich in omega-3s and fiber)
- Berries (high in antioxidants and fiber)
- Limited added sugar (optional)

Note: You can also make this recipe overnight by soaking the oats and chia seeds in the almond milk in the refrigerator for at least 4 hours or overnight, then topping with berries and other toppings in the morning.

2. Avocado Toast With Poached Eggs

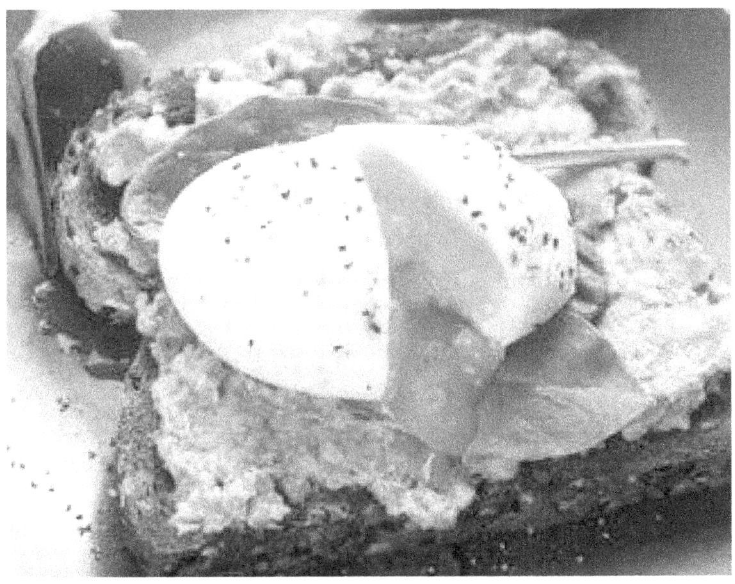

Ingredients:
- 2 slices whole grain bread
- 1 ripe avocado, mashed
- 2 poached eggs
- Salt and pepper to taste
- Optional: cherry tomatoes, spinach, feta cheese, red pepper flakes

Instructions:
1. Toast the bread until lightly browned.
2. Spread the mashed avocado on top of the toast.
3. Poach the eggs and place them on top of the avocado.

4. Season with salt and pepper to taste.
5. Add optional toppings if desired.

Tips:
- Use whole grain bread for a fiber and nutrient boost.
- Add a squeeze of lemon juice to the avocado for extra flavor.
- Top with cherry tomatoes for a burst of juicy sweetness.
- Add a sprinkle of red pepper flakes for a spicy kick.
- Use a fried egg or scrambled eggs if you prefer.

This recipe is PCOS-friendly because it includes:

- Whole grains (bread)
- Healthy fats (avocado)
- Protein (eggs)
- Fiber and antioxidants (optional cherry tomatoes and spinach)

Note: You can also make this recipe into a breakfast sandwich by adding a slice of whole grain bread on top and wrapping it in a napkin for a portable breakfast on-the-go.

3. Greek Yogurt Parfait With Granola And Berries

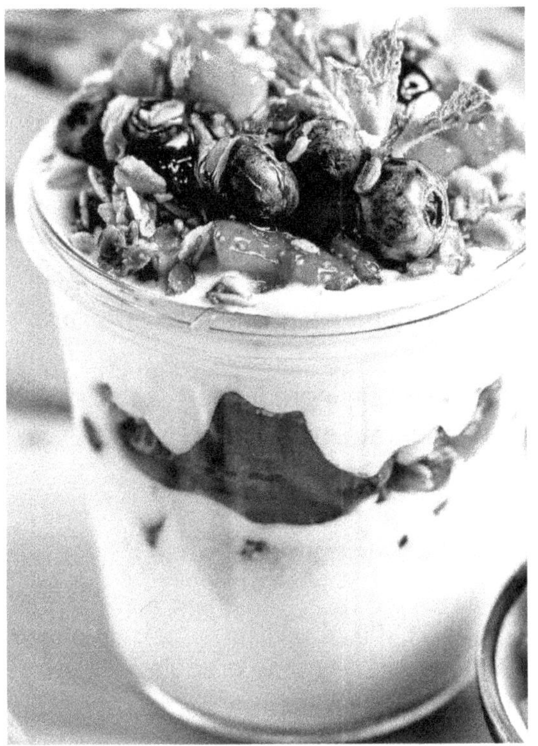

Ingredients:

- 1 cup Greek yogurt
- 1/4 cup granola
- 1 cup mixed berries (fresh or frozen)
- 1 tablespoon honey or maple syrup (optional)
- 1/4 teaspoon vanilla extract (optional)

Instructions:

1. Layer the yogurt, granola, and berries in a bowl.

2. Drizzle with honey or maple syrup and add vanilla extract if using.
3. Serve chilled and enjoy!

Tips:
- Use a high-protein Greek yogurt for an extra boost.
- Choose a low-sugar granola or make your own with nuts and seeds.
- Mix and match different types of berries, such as blueberries, strawberries, and raspberries.
- Add a sprinkle of cinnamon or nutmeg for extra flavor.
- Make ahead: Layer the ingredients in a jar or container and refrigerate overnight for a quick breakfast or snack.

This recipe is PCOS-friendly because it includes:
- Protein-rich Greek yogurt
- Fiber and healthy fats from the granola
- Antioxidant-rich berries
- Limited added sugar (optional)

Note: You can also customize this recipe with other toppings, such as sliced almonds, shredded coconut, or diced mango.

4. Smoothie Bowl With Spinach, Banana, And Almond Milk

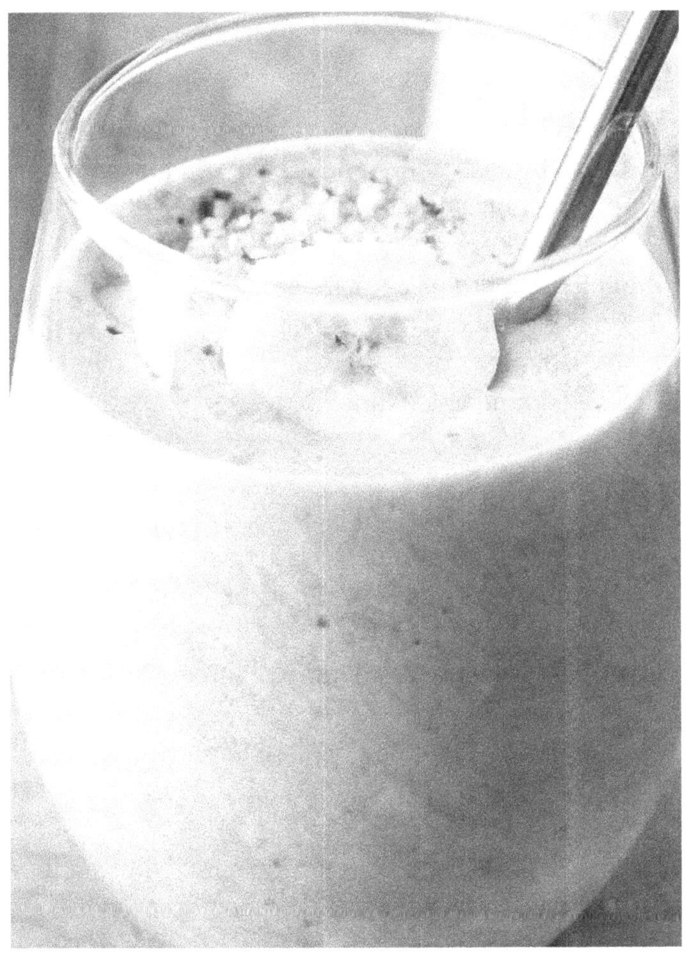

Ingredients:
- 2 cups spinach
- 1 ripe banana
- 1 cup almond milk

- 1/2 cup frozen pineapple
- 1 tablespoon chia seeds
- 1 scoop protein powder (optional)
- Toppings: sliced fruit, granola, coconut flakes, nut butter

Instructions:

1. Blend the spinach, banana, almond milk, and pineapple until smooth.
2. Add the chia seeds and protein powder (if using) and blend until well combined.
3. Pour into a bowl and top with your favorite ingredients.
4. Serve immediately and enjoy.

Tips:

- Use fresh or frozen spinach - both work
- Add a squeeze of fresh lime juice for extra flavor.
- Substitute other non-dairy milk alternatives like soy milk or coconut milk.
- Add a sprinkle of cinnamon or nutmeg for extra flavor.
- Make ahead: Blend the smoothie and store in the fridge for up to 24 hours, then top and serve.

Note: You can also customize this recipe with other ingredients, such as mango, berries, or peanut butter.

5. Whole Grain Waffles With Fresh Fruit And Yogurt

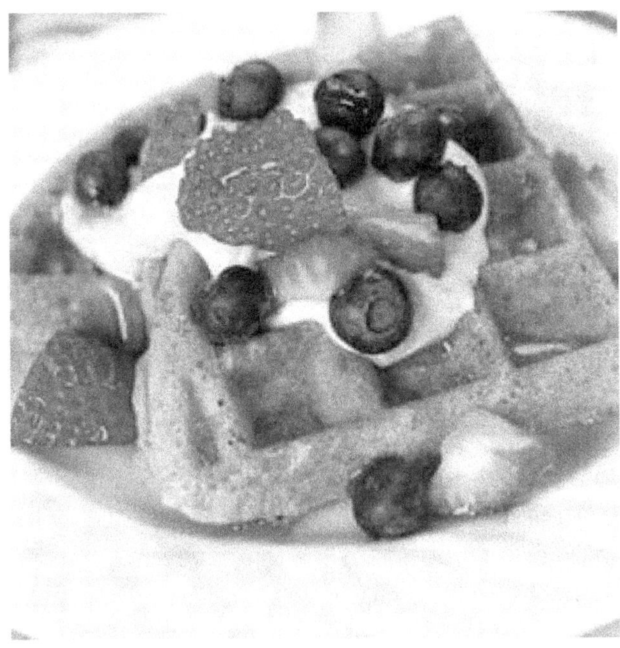

Ingredients:
- 2 cups whole grain flour
- 4 teaspoons baking powder
- 1 teaspoon salt
- 1 cup unsweetened almond milk
- 1 large egg
- 2 tablespoons melted coconut oil
- Fresh fruit (such as berries, sliced banana, or diced mango)
- Yogurt (plain or flavored)

Instructions:

1. Preheat waffle iron according to manufacturer's instructions.
2. In a large bowl, whisk together flour, baking powder, and salt.
3. In a separate bowl, whisk together almond milk, egg, and melted coconut oil.
4. Pour wet ingredients into dry ingredients and stir until just combined.
5. Pour batter into waffle iron and cook until golden brown.
6. Serve with fresh fruit and yogurt.

Tips:
- Use a high-protein whole grain flour for an extra boost.
- Add a sprinkle of cinnamon or nutmeg to the batter for extra flavor.
- Use different types of milk alternatives, such as soy milk or coconut milk.
- Top with a drizzle of honey or maple syrup for a touch of sweetness.
- Make ahead: Cook waffles and store in the fridge for up to 3 days or freeze for up to 2 months.

Note: You can also customize this recipe with other toppings, such as granola, chopped nuts, or seeds.

6. Veggie Omelette With Whole Grain Toast

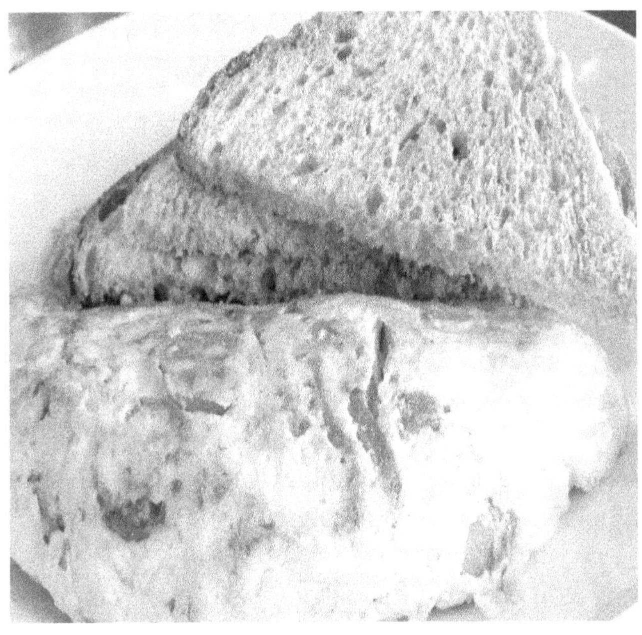

Ingredients:
- 2 eggs
- 1/2 cup diced bell peppers
- 1/2 cup diced onions
- 1/2 cup diced mushrooms
- 2 cloves garlic, minced
- 1 tablespoon olive oil
- Salt and pepper to taste
- 2 slices whole grain bread
- Optional: shredded cheese, salsa, avocado

Instructions:

1. In a bowl, whisk together eggs and a pinch of salt.
2. Heat olive oil in a skillet over medium heat.
3. Add diced veggies and cook until tender.
4. Pour in eggs and cook until set.
5. Fold the omelet in half and cook for another minute.
6. Serve with whole grain toast and optional toppings.

Tips:
- Use any combination of veggies you like!
- Add a sprinkle of feta cheese for extra flavor.
- Use a non-stick skillet for easy egg cooking.
- Make ahead: Cook veggies and eggs, then assemble the omelet just before serving.
- Whole grain toast provides fiber and B vitamins.

Note: You can also customize this recipe with other fillings, such as diced ham or spinach.

7. Chia Seed Pudding With Coconut Milk And Fresh Fruit

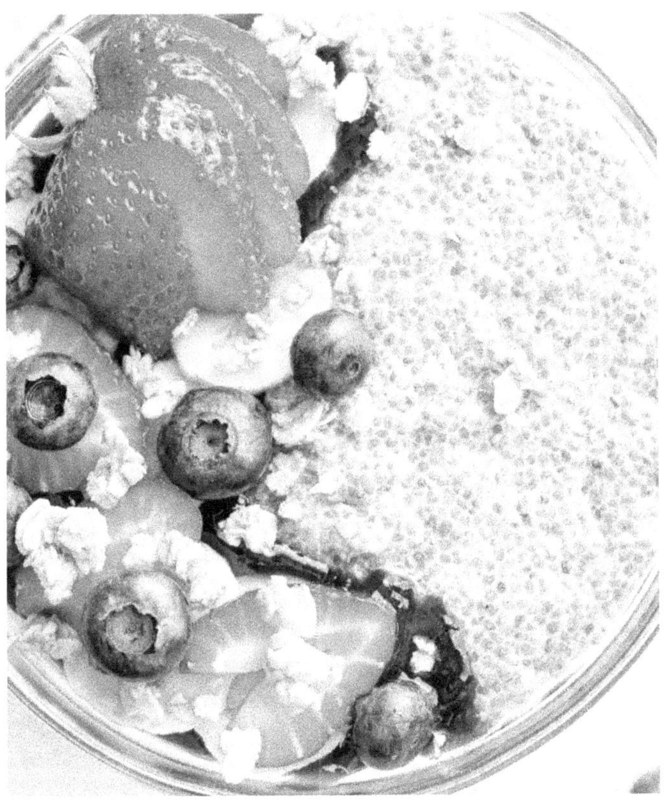

Ingredients:
- 1/2 cup chia seeds
- 1 cup coconut milk
- 1 tablespoon honey or maple syrup (optional)
- 1/4 teaspoon vanilla extract (optional)
- Fresh fruit (such as berries, sliced mango, or diced pineapple)

Instructions:
1. In a bowl, mix together chia seeds, coconut milk, honey or maple syrup (if using), and vanilla extract (if using).
2. Refrigerate for at least 2 hours or overnight until chia seeds are gelatinous.
3. Top with fresh fruit and serve.

Tips:
- Use full-fat coconut milk for the creamiest texture.
- Add a sprinkle of cinnamon or nutmeg for extra flavor.
- Mix in other ingredients like cocoa powder or matcha powder for different flavors.
- Make ahead: Prepare chia seed pudding and store in the fridge for up to 5 days.
- Chia seeds provide omega-3s and fiber.

Note: You can also customize this recipe with other toppings, such as granola or shredded coconut.

8. Cottage Cheese With Sliced Peaches And Cinnamon

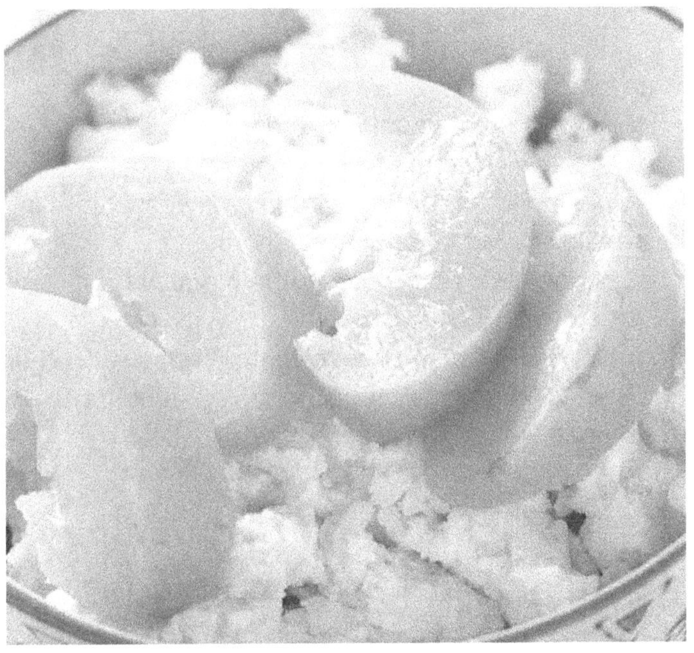

Ingredients:
- 1 cup cottage cheese
- 1/2 cup sliced peaches
- 1/4 teaspoon ground cinnamon
- 1 tablespoon honey or maple syrup (optional)

Instructions:
1. In a bowl, mix together cottage cheese, sliced peaches, and cinnamon.
2. Add honey or maple syrup (if using) and mix well.
3. Serve immediately and enjoy!

Tips:
- Use low-sodium cottage cheese to reduce salt intake.
- Add a sprinkle of nutmeg or cardamom for extra flavor.
- Mix in other ingredients like berries or sliced bananas for different flavors.
- Make ahead: Prepare cottage cheese mixture and store in the fridge for up to 24 hours.
- Cottage cheese provides protein and calcium.

Note: You can also customize this recipe with other toppings, such as sliced almonds or shredded coconut.

9. Green Smoothie With Spinach, Banana, And Protein Powder

Ingredients:
- 2 cups spinach
- 1 ripe banana
- 1 scoop protein powder
- 1 cup unsweetened almond milk
- 1/2 cup frozen pineapple
- 1 tablespoon chia seeds
- 1 teaspoon honey or maple syrup (optional)

Instructions:
1. Blend all ingredients In a blender until smooth.

2. Add honey or maple syrup (if using) and blend well.

3. Pour into a glass and serve immediately.

Tips:

- Use fresh or frozen spinach - both work great!

- Add a squeeze of fresh lime juice for extra flavor.

- Substitute other non-dairy milk alternatives like soy milk or coconut milk.

- Add a sprinkle of cinnamon or nutmeg for extra flavor.

- Make ahead: Blend smoothies and store in the fridge for up to 24 hours.

10. Turkey And Avocado Wrap With Mixed Greens

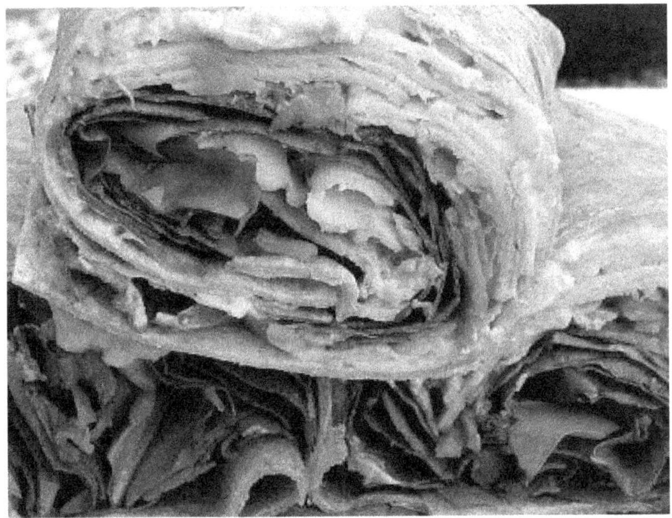

Ingredients:

- 1 whole wheat tortilla
- 2 slices deli turkey breast
- 1/2 avocado, sliced
- 1 cup mixed greens
- 1/4 cup sliced cucumber
- 1/4 cup sliced bell peppers
- 1 tablespoon hummus

Instructions:

1. Lay the tortilla flat and arrange ingredients in the center.
2. Fold bottom half up, then fold in sides and roll up tightly.
3. Slice in half and serve.

Tips:

- Use whole wheat tortillas for extra fiber.
- Add a sprinkle of feta cheese for extra flavor.
- Substitute other protein sources like chicken or tofu.
- Add a drizzle of balsamic glaze for extra flavor.
- Make ahead: Prepare ingredients and assemble wrap just before serving.

11. Quinoa Salad With Roasted Vegetables And Lemon Vinaigrette

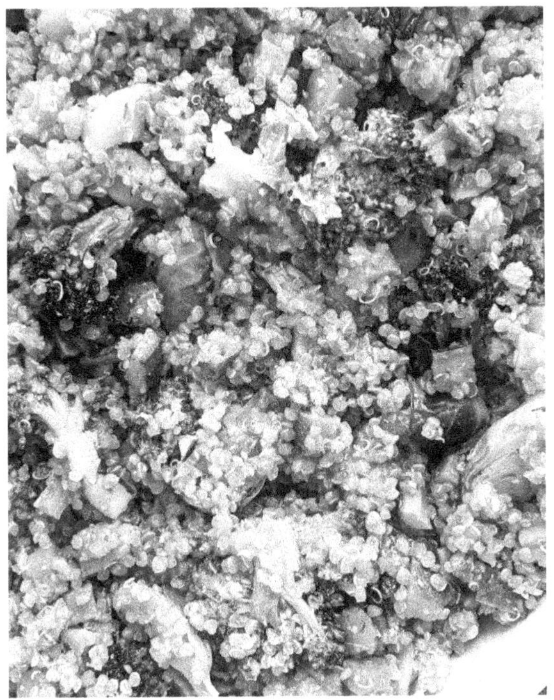

Ingredients:

- 1 cup cooked quinoa
- 2 cups mixed roasted vegetables (such as sweet potatoes, Brussels sprouts, and red onions)
- 1/4 cup freshly squeezed lemon juice
- 2 tablespoons olive oil
- 1 teaspoon Dijon mustard
- Salt and pepper to taste
- Fresh parsley or cilantro (optional)

Instructions:

1. In a large bowl, combine quinoa and roasted vegetables.
2. In a small bowl, whisk together lemon juice, olive oil, and Dijon mustard.
3. Pour dressing over quinoa mixture and toss to coat.
4. Season with salt and pepper to taste.
5. Garnish with fresh parsley or cilantro (if using).

Tips:

- Use pre-cooked quinoa to save time.
- Customize with your favorite roasted vegetables.
- Add a sprinkle of feta cheese for extra flavor.
- Make ahead: Prepare quinoa and roasted vegetables, then assemble salad just before serving.

12. Grilled Chicken And Vegetable Skewers With Chimichurri Sauce

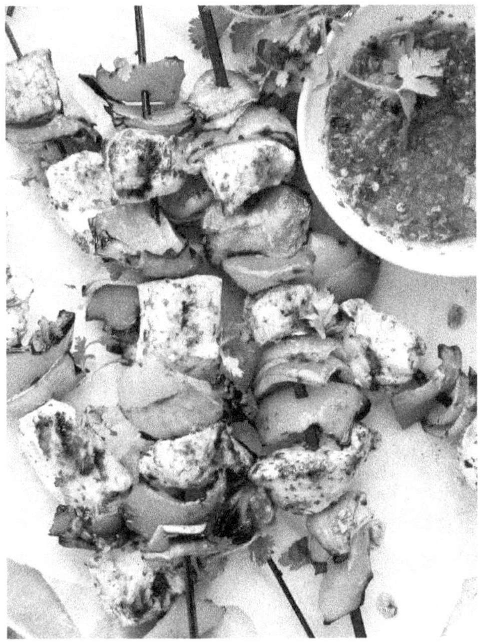

Ingredients:
- 1 pound boneless, skinless chicken breast, cut into bite-sized pieces
- 1 cup mixed vegetables, such as cherry tomatoes, bell peppers, onions, and mushrooms
- 1/4 cup fresh parsley, chopped
- 1/4 cup fresh oregano, chopped
- 2 cloves garlic, minced
- 1/4 cup red wine vinegar
- 1/4 cup olive oil

- Salt and pepper to taste

Instructions:
1. Preheat the grill to medium-high heat.
2. Thread chicken and vegetables onto skewers.
3. In a bowl, mix together parsley, oregano, garlic, red wine vinegar, and olive oil.
4. Brush chimichurri sauce onto skewers.
5. Grill for 10-12 minutes, or until chicken is cooked through.
6. Serve with additional chimichurri sauce for dipping.

Tips:
- Use any combination of vegetables you like.
- Add a sprinkle of feta cheese for extra flavor.
- Make ahead: Prepare skewers and chimichurri sauce, then grill just before serving.

13. Lentil Soup With Spinach And Feta

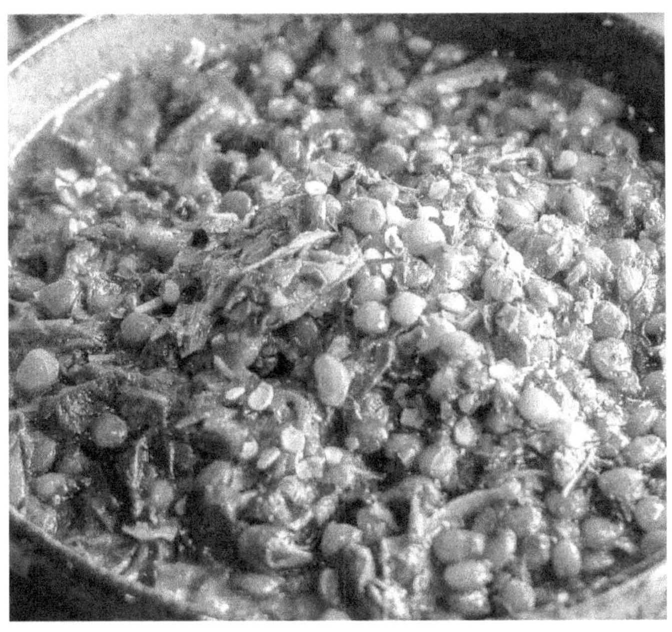

Ingredients:
- 1 cup dried green or brown lentils, rinsed and drained
- 4 cups vegetable broth
- 1 onion, chopped
- 2 cloves garlic, minced
- 1 carrot, chopped
- 1 celery stalk, chopped
- 1 can diced tomatoes
- 1/4 cup chopped fresh spinach
- 2 tablespoons olive oil
- 1/2 cup crumbled feta cheese (optional)

- Salt and pepper to taste

Instructions:
1. In a pot, sauté onion, garlic, carrot, and celery in olive oil until tender.
2. Add lentils, vegetable broth, and diced tomatoes. Bring to a boil, then reduce heat and simmer for 30-40 minutes, or until lentils are tender.
3. Stir in spinach and cook until wilted.
4. Season with salt and pepper to taste.
5. Serve with crumbled feta cheese on top (if using).

Tips:
- Use red or yellow lentils for a different flavor and texture.
- Add a sprinkle of paprika or cumin for extra flavor.
- Make ahead: Prepare soup and refrigerate or freeze for up to 3 days.
- Lentils provide protein, fiber, and minerals like iron and potassium.

Note: You can also customize this recipe with other ingredients, such as chopped bell peppers or a squeeze of lemon juice.

14. Grilled Salmon With Roasted Asparagus And Brown Rice

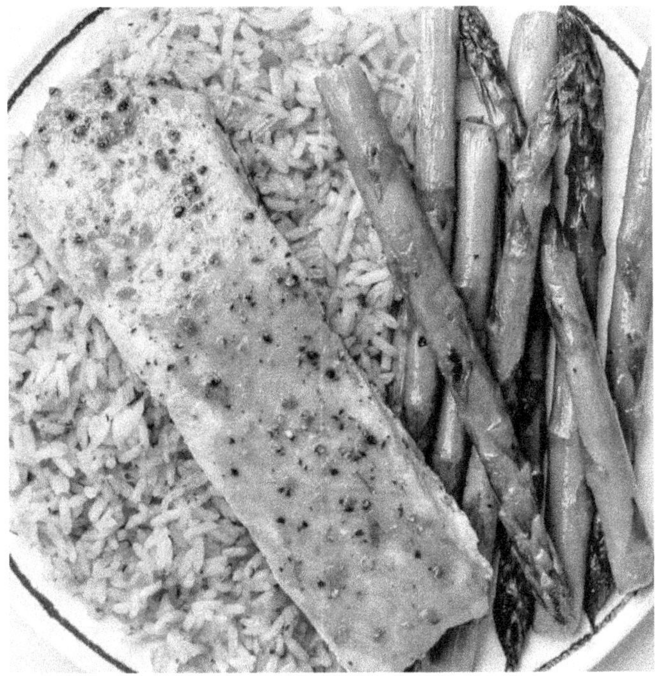

Ingredients:
- 4 salmon filets (6 ounces each)
- 1 pound fresh asparagus, trimmed
- 2 cups cooked brown rice
- 2 tablespoons olive oil
- Salt and pepper to taste
- Optional: lemon wedges, chopped fresh parsley

Instructions:
1. Preheat the grill to medium-high heat.

2. Season salmon with salt and pepper. Grill for 4-6 minutes per side, or until cooked through.
3. Toss asparagus with olive oil, salt, and pepper. Spread on a baking sheet and roast in the oven at 425°F for 12-15 minutes, or until tender.
4. Serve salmon with roasted asparagus and brown rice.
5. Garnish with lemon wedges and chopped parsley (if using).

Tips:
- Use wild-caught salmon for higher nutritional value.
- Add a squeeze of fresh lemon juice for extra flavor.
- Make ahead: Prepare brown rice and roast asparagus ahead of time.
- Salmon provides omega-3 fatty acids, while asparagus is rich in vitamin C and folate.

15. Stuffed Bell Peppers With Quinoa, Black Beans, And Cheese

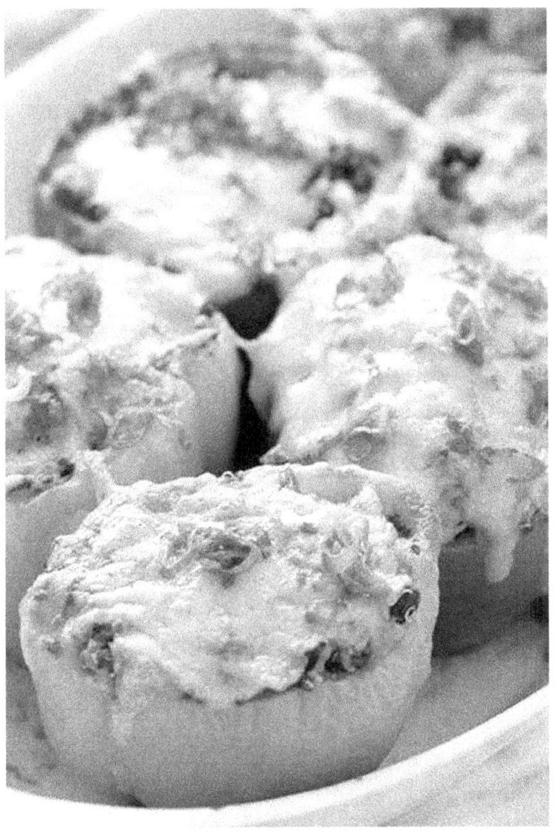

Ingredients:
- 4 bell peppers, any color
- 1 cup cooked quinoa
- 1 cup cooked black beans
- 1 cup shredded cheese (Monterey Jack or Cheddar)

- 1/2 cup chopped fresh cilantro
- 1 lime, juiced
- 1 teaspoon cumin
- Salt and pepper to taste

Instructions:
1. Preheat the oven to 375°F.
2. Cut tops off bell peppers and remove seeds and membranes.
3. In a bowl, mix together quinoa, black beans, cheese, cilantro, lime juice, and cumin.
4. Stuff each bell pepper with the quinoa mixture and top with the pepper top.
5. Bake for 25-30 minutes, or until bell peppers are tender.

Tips:
- Use any color bell pepper you like!
- Add a sprinkle of paprika for extra flavor.
- Make ahead: Prepare quinoa mixture and stuff bell peppers, then bake just before serving.
- Quinoa provides protein and fiber, while black beans add folate and magnesium.

Delicious Lunch Recipes

1. Grilled Chicken And Veggie Wrap With Hummus

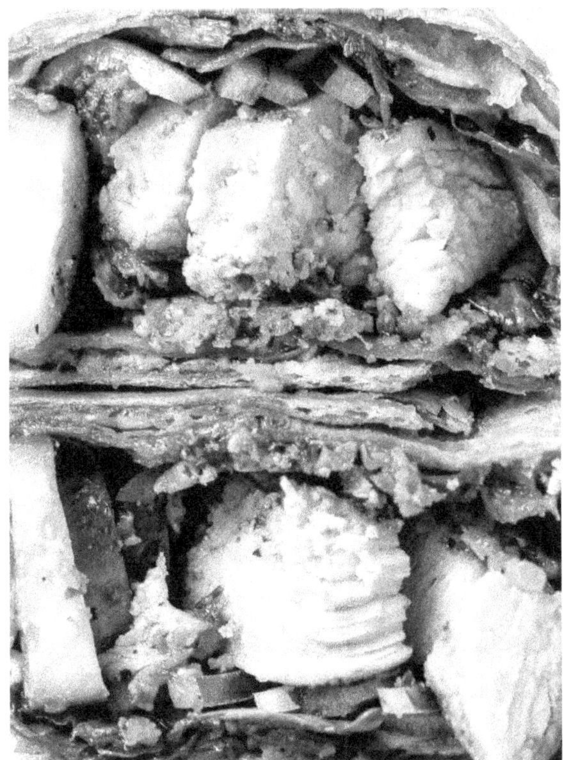

Ingredients:
- 1 boneless, skinless chicken breast
- 1/2 cup hummus
- 1 large flour tortilla
- 1 cup mixed greens

- 1 cup sliced veggies (bell peppers, cucumber, carrots)
- 1/4 cup sliced red onion
- 1/4 cup crumbled feta cheese (optional)

Instructions:
1. Grill the chicken breast and slice into strips.
2. Spread hummus on the tortilla.
3. Add the mixed greens, sliced veggies, and chicken strips.
4. Top with red onion and feta cheese (if using).
5. Roll up the wrap and slice in half.

Tips:
- Use whole wheat tortillas for extra fiber.
- Add a sprinkle of paprika for extra flavor.
- Make ahead: Prepare the chicken and veggies, then assemble the wrap just before serving.

2. Quinoa And Black Bean Salad With Avocado Dressing

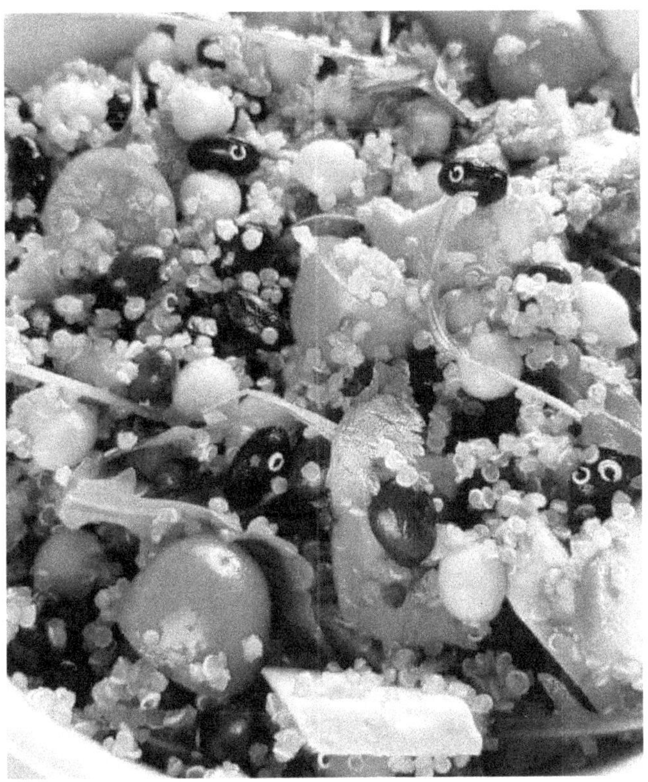

Ingredients:

- 1 cup cooked quinoa
- 1 cup cooked black beans
- 1 cup diced veggies (bell peppers, onions, tomatoes)
- 1/2 cup chopped fresh cilantro
- 2 tablespoons lime juice
- 1 ripe avocado, diced

- Salt and pepper to taste

Instructions:
1. In a large bowl, mix together quinoa, black beans, veggies, and cilantro.
2. In a separate bowl, mix together lime juice and avocado.
3. Pour the avocado dressing over the quinoa mixture and toss to coat.
4. Season with salt and pepper to taste.

Tips:
- Use any color bell pepper you like!
- Add a sprinkle of cumin for extra flavor.
- Make ahead: Prepare the quinoa and black bean mixture, then assemble the salad just before serving.

3. Grilled Salmon And Brown Rice Bowl With Roasted Veggies

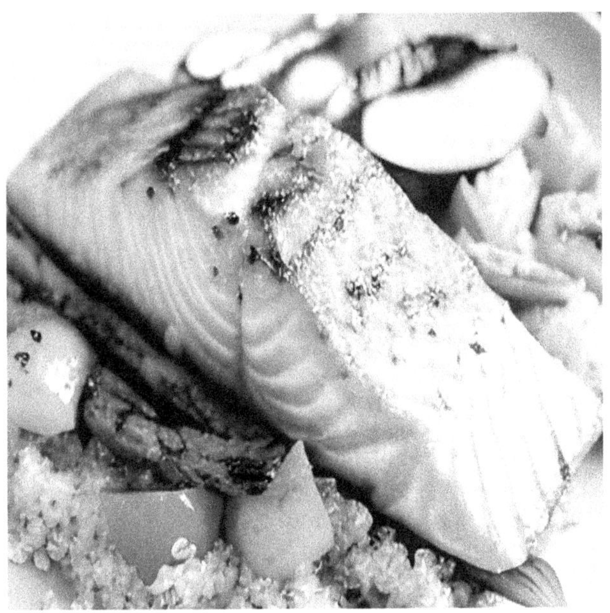

Ingredients:
- 4 salmon filets (6 ounces each)
- 1 cup brown rice
- 2 cups water
- 2 tablespoons olive oil
- 1 large sweet potato, peeled and cubed
- 1 large zucchini, sliced
- 1 large red bell pepper, sliced
- Salt and pepper to taste
- Optional: lemon wedges, chopped fresh parsley

Instructions:
1. Preheat the grill to medium-high heat.

2. Cook brown rice according to package instructions.
3. Grill salmon for 4-6 minutes per side, or until cooked through.
4. Toss sweet potato, zucchini, and red bell pepper with olive oil, salt, and pepper. Spread on a baking sheet and roast in the oven at 425°F for 20-25 minutes, or until tender.
5. Serve salmon on top of brown rice with roasted veggies and a squeeze of lemon juice (if using). Garnish with parsley (if using).

Tips:
- Use wild-caught salmon for higher nutritional value.
- Add a sprinkle of paprika for extra flavor.
- Make ahead: Prepare brown rice and roast veggies ahead of time.

4. Turkey and Avocado Salad With Mixed Greens And Lemon Vinaigrette

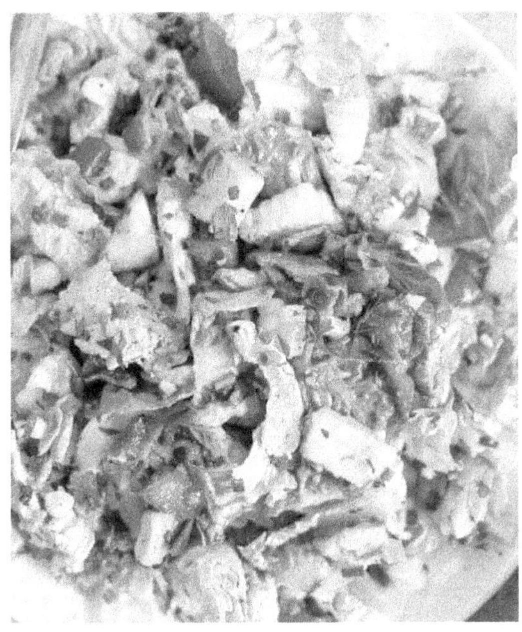

Ingredients:
- 4 ounces sliced turkey breast
- 1 ripe avocado, diced
- 4 cups mixed greens
- 1 cup cherry tomatoes, halved
- 1/2 cup sliced red onion
- 2 tablespoons freshly squeezed lemon juice
- 1 tablespoon olive oil
- Salt and pepper to taste

Instructions:

1. In a large bowl, combine mixed greens, turkey, avocado, cherry tomatoes, and red onion.
2. In a small bowl, whisk together lemon juice and olive oil.
3. Pour the dressing over the salad and toss to coat.
4. Season with salt and pepper to taste.

Tips:
- Use whole wheat tortillas for extra fiber.
- Add a sprinkle of feta cheese for extra flavor.
- Make ahead: Prepare the salad and dressing separately, then assemble just before serving.

5. Chickpea And Spinach Curry With Brown Rice

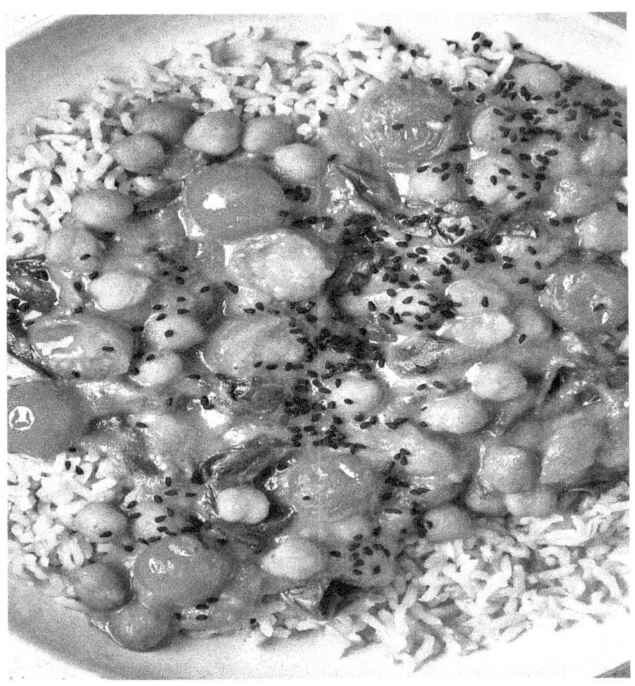

Ingredients:
- 1 can chickpeas
- 2 cups fresh spinach
- 2 cups water
- 1 onion, chopped
- 2 cloves garlic, minced
- 1 tablespoon curry powder
- 1 teaspoon turmeric
- 1/2 teaspoon cumin
- 1/2 teaspoon paprika
- Salt and pepper to taste

- 2 tablespoons olive oil
- 1 cup brown rice

Instructions:
1. Cook brown rice according to package instructions.
2. In a pot, sauté onion, garlic, curry powder, turmeric, cumin, paprika, and chickpeas in olive oil until fragrant.
3. Add water and bring to a boil, then reduce heat and simmer for 10-15 minutes.
4. Stir in spinach and cook until wilted.
5. Serve curry over brown rice.

Tips:
- Use fresh spinach for the best flavor and nutrition.
- Add a squeeze of fresh lime juice for extra flavor.
- Make ahead: Prepare curry and rice separately, then assemble just before serving.

6. Zucchini Boats With Turkey And Feta Filling

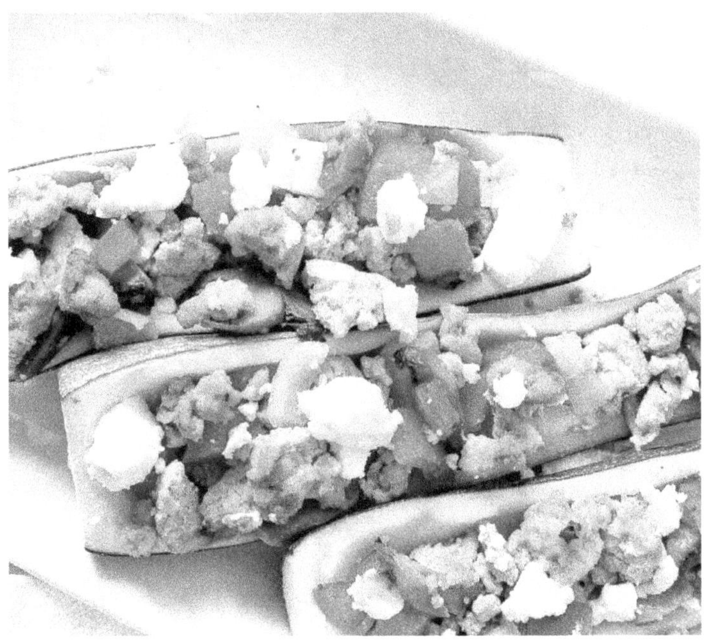

Ingredients:
- 4 medium zucchinis
- 1 pound ground turkey
- 1/2 cup crumbled feta cheese
- 1/4 cup chopped fresh parsley
- 2 cloves garlic, minced
- 1 tablespoon olive oil
- Salt and pepper to taste

Instructions:
1. Preheat the oven to 375°F.
2. Scoop out zucchini flesh, leaving a shell.

3. In a bowl, mix together turkey, feta, parsley, garlic, and olive oil.
4. Stuff each zucchini boat with the turkey mixture.
5. Bake for 25-30 minutes, or until zucchinis are tender.

Tips:
- Use lean ground turkey for a healthier option.
- Add a sprinkle of paprika for extra flavor.
- Make ahead: Prepare filling and scoop out zucchinis ahead of time.

7. Grilled Chicken And Strawberry Salad With Feta And Balsamic Glaze

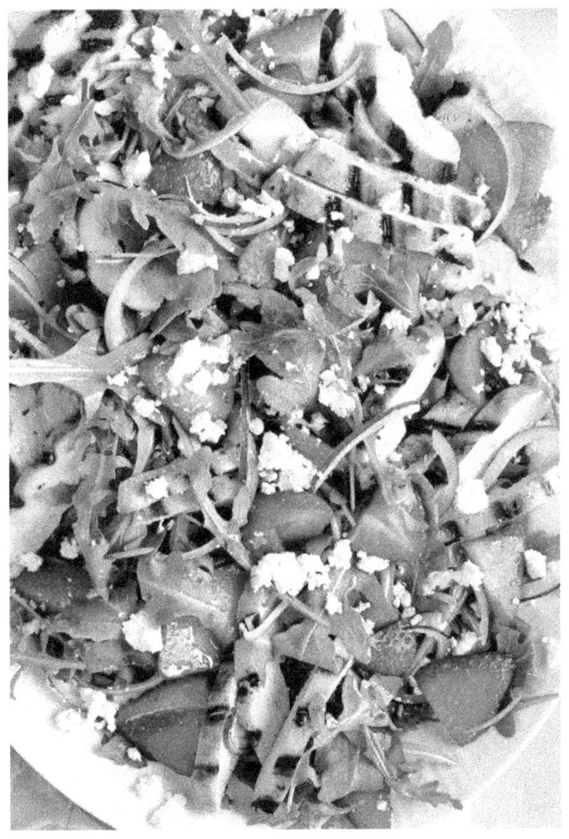

Ingredients:

- 4 boneless, skinless chicken breasts
- 2 cups mixed greens
- 1 pint fresh strawberries, sliced
- 1/2 cup crumbled feta cheese

- 1/4 cup chopped fresh mint
- 2 tablespoons balsamic glaze
- 1 tablespoon olive oil
- Salt and pepper to taste

Instructions:

1. Grill chicken breasts until cooked through.
2. In a large bowl, combine mixed greens, strawberries, feta, and mint.
3. Slice grilled chicken and add to the salad.
4. Drizzle with balsamic glaze and olive oil.
5. Season with salt and pepper to taste.

Tips:

- Use fresh strawberries for the best flavor and nutrition.
- Add a sprinkle of chopped pecans for extra crunch.
- Make ahead: Prepare salad and grill chicken ahead of time.

8. Veggie And Bean Chili With Quinoa And Greek Yogurt

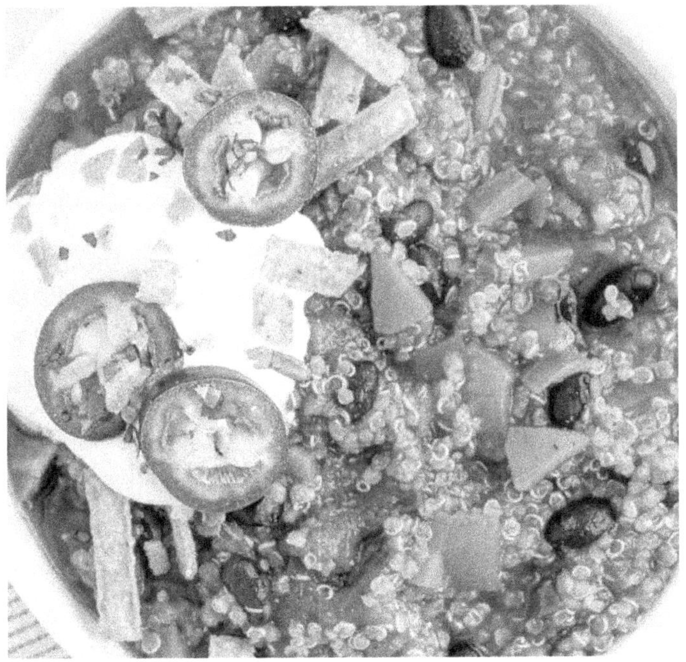

Ingredients:
- 1 cup quinoa
- 2 cups water
- 1 can black beans, drained and rinsed
- 1 can diced tomatoes
- 1 onion, chopped
- 2 cloves garlic, minced
- 1 red bell pepper, chopped
- 1 can corn, drained
- 1 tablespoon chili powder
- 1 teaspoon cumin

- Salt and pepper to taste
- 6 ounces Greek yogurt (optional)

Instructions:
1. Cook quinoa according to package instructions.
2. In a pot, sauté onion, garlic, and red bell pepper until tender.
3. Add chili powder, cumin, black beans, diced tomatoes, and corn. Simmer for 20-25 minutes.
4. Serve chili over quinoa.
5. Top with Greek yogurt, if desired.

Tips:
- Use any color bell pepper you like!
- Add a sprinkle of paprika for extra flavor.
- Make ahead: Prepare chili and quinoa ahead of time.

9. Tuna Salad Sandwich With Mixed Greens And Whole Wheat Bread

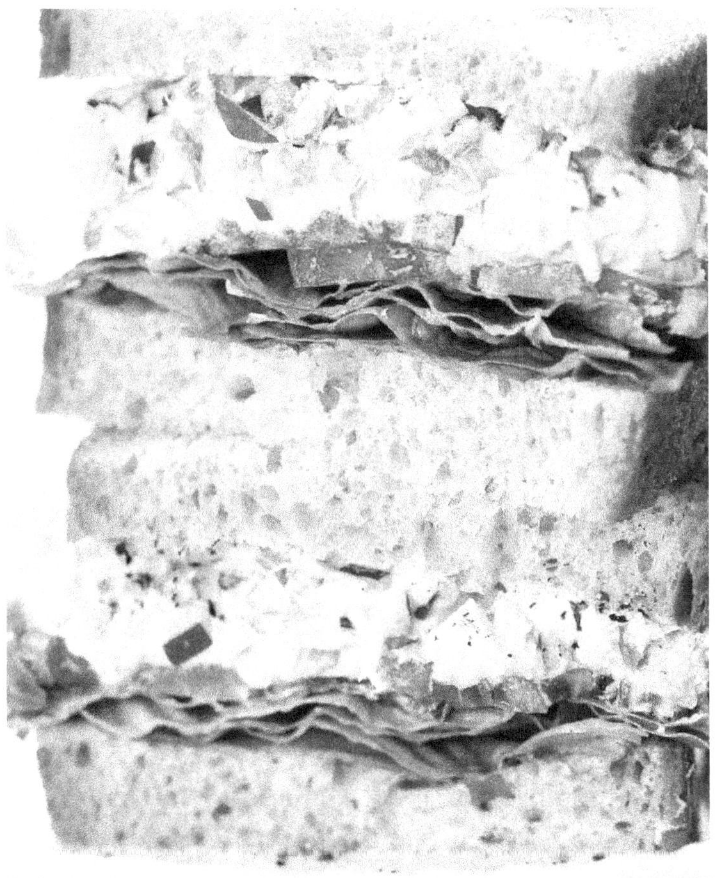

Ingredients:
- 1 can tuna (drained and flaked)
- 1/4 cup mayonnaise
- 1/4 cup chopped celery

- 1/4 cup chopped red onion
- 1/4 cup chopped fresh parsley
- Salt and pepper to taste
- 4 slices whole wheat bread
- 4 cups mixed greens
- 2 tablespoons olive oil
- 1 tablespoon lemon juice

Instructions:

1. In a bowl, mix together tuna, mayonnaise, celery, onion, and parsley.
2. Season with salt and pepper to taste.
3. Divide tuna salad among four slices of whole wheat bread.
4. Top with mixed greens and drizzle with olive oil and lemon juice.

Tips:

- Use low-mercury tuna for a healthier option.
- Add a sprinkle of paprika for extra flavor.
- Make ahead: Prepare tuna salad and store in the refrigerator for up to 3 days.

10. Roasted Vegetable And Brown Rice Bowl With Grilled Chicken

Ingredients:

- 1 cup brown rice
- 2 cups water
- 2 boneless, skinless chicken breasts

- 2 tablespoons olive oil
- 1 large sweet potato, peeled and cubed
- 1 large carrot, peeled and sliced
- 1 large zucchini, sliced
- 1 large red bell pepper, seeded and sliced
- Salt and pepper to taste

Instructions:
1. Preheat the oven to 425°F.
2. Cook brown rice according to package instructions.
3. Grill chicken breasts until cooked through.
4. Toss sweet potato, carrot, zucchini, and red bell pepper with olive oil, salt, and pepper. Spread on a baking sheet and roast in the oven for 25-30 minutes, or until tender.
5. Serve grilled chicken on top of brown rice with roasted vegetables.

Tips:
- Use any color bell pepper you like!
- Add a sprinkle of paprika for extra flavor.
- Make ahead: Prepare brown rice and roast vegetables ahead of time.

11. Spinach And Feta Stuffed Chicken Breast With Roasted Asparagus

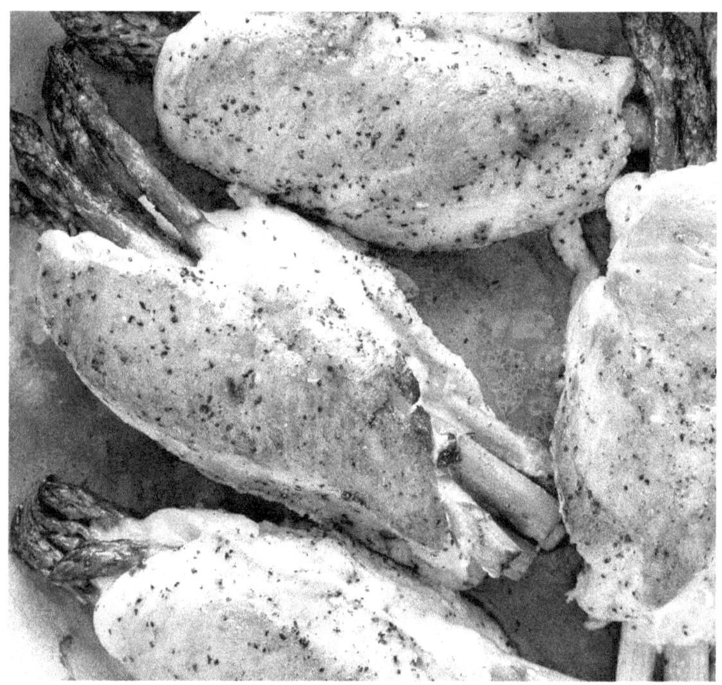

Ingredients:

- 4 boneless, skinless chicken breasts
- 1 package frozen chopped spinach, thawed and drained
- 1/2 cup crumbled feta cheese
- 2 cloves garlic, minced
- 1 tablespoon olive oil
- Salt and pepper to taste
- 1 pound fresh asparagus, trimmed

Instructions:
1. Preheat the oven to 375°F.
2. In a bowl, mix together spinach, feta, garlic, and olive oil.
3. Stuff each chicken breast with the spinach mixture and bake for 25-30 minutes, or until cooked through.
4. Toss asparagus with olive oil, salt, and pepper. Spread on a baking sheet and roast in the oven for 12-15 minutes, or until tender.
5. Serve chicken breasts with roasted asparagus.

Tips:
- Use fresh spinach for the best flavor and nutrition.
- Add a sprinkle of paprika for extra flavor.
- Make ahead: Prepare spinach mixture and stuff chicken breasts ahead of time.

12. Lentil And Vegetable Curry With Brown Rice

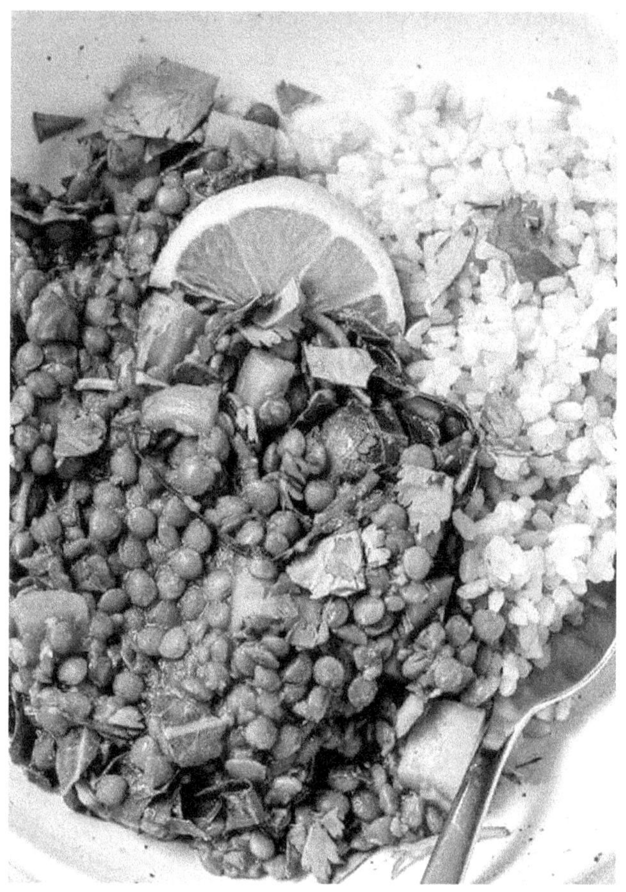

Ingredients:
- 1 cup brown rice
- 2 cups water
- 1 cup red or green lentils, rinsed and drained
- 2 cups water
- 1 onion, chopped

- 2 cloves garlic, minced
- 1 carrot, chopped
- 1 zucchini, chopped
- 1 red bell pepper, chopped
- 1 can diced tomatoes
- 1 tablespoon curry powder
- 1 teaspoon turmeric
- Salt and pepper to taste

Instructions:

1. Cook brown rice according to package instructions.
2. In a pot, sauté onion, garlic, carrot, zucchini, and red bell pepper until tender.
3. Add lentils, water, diced tomatoes, curry powder, turmeric, salt, and pepper. Bring to a boil, then reduce heat and simmer for 20-25 minutes, or until lentils are tender.
4. Serve curry over brown rice.

Tips:

- Use any color bell pepper you like.
- Add a sprinkle of paprika for extra flavor.
- Make ahead: Prepare curry and rice ahead of time.

13. Grilled Salmon With Roasted Vegetables And Quinoa

Ingredients:

- 4 salmon filets (6 ounces each)
- 1 cup quinoa
- 2 cups water
- 2 tablespoons olive oil
- 1 large sweet potato, peeled and cubed
- 1 large zucchini, sliced
- 1 large red bell pepper, seeded and sliced
- Salt and pepper to taste

Instructions:
1. Preheat the grill to medium-high heat.
2. Cook quinoa according to package instructions.
3. Grill salmon filets for 4-6 minutes per side, or until cooked through.
4. Toss sweet potato, zucchini, and red bell pepper with olive oil, salt, and pepper. Spread on a baking sheet and roast in the oven for 20-25 minutes, or until tender.
5. Serve grilled salmon with roasted vegetables and quinoa.

Tips:
- Use any color bell pepper you like!
- Add a sprinkle of paprika for extra flavor.
- Make ahead: Prepare quinoa and roast vegetables ahead of time.

14. Grilled Chicken And Salad

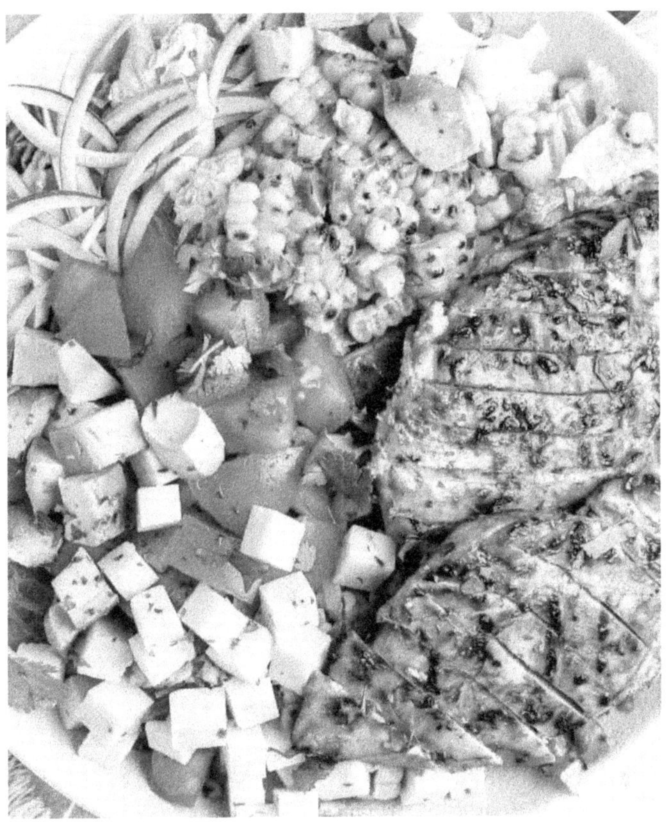

Grilled Chicken
Ingredients:
- 4 boneless, skinless chicken breasts
- 2 tbsp olive oil
- 1 tsp lemon juice
- 1 tsp garlic powder
- Salt and pepper to taste

Instructions:

1. Preheat the grill to medium-high heat.
2. In a small bowl, whisk together olive oil, lemon juice, garlic powder, salt, and pepper.
3. Brush the mixture on both sides of the chicken breasts.
4. Grill for 5-6 minutes per side or until cooked through.
5. Let rest for a few minutes before slicing.

Salad
Ingredients:
- 4 cups mixed greens (arugula, spinach, lettuce)
- 1 cup cherry tomatoes, halved
- 1 cup sliced cucumber
- 1/2 cup sliced red onion
- 1/4 cup crumbled feta cheese (optional)
- 1/4 cup chopped fresh parsley
- 2 tbsp olive oil
- 1 tbsp lemon juice
- Salt and pepper to taste

Instructions:
1. In a large bowl, combine mixed greens, cherry tomatoes, cucumber, red onion, and feta cheese (if using).
2. In a small bowl, whisk together olive oil and lemon juice.
3. Pour the dressing over the salad and toss to combine.
4. Sprinkle parsley on top and serve with sliced grilled chicken.

Tips:
- Choose lean protein sources like chicken breast, which is low in saturated fat and high in protein.
- Include plenty of fiber-rich vegetables like mixed greens, cherry tomatoes, and cucumber.
- Healthy fats like olive oil and avocado (optional) support hormone balance and satiety.
- Limit or avoid added sugars, refined carbohydrates, and processed foods.

15. Grilled Shrimp And Pineapple Skewers With Spicy Mango Sauce And Cauliflower Rice

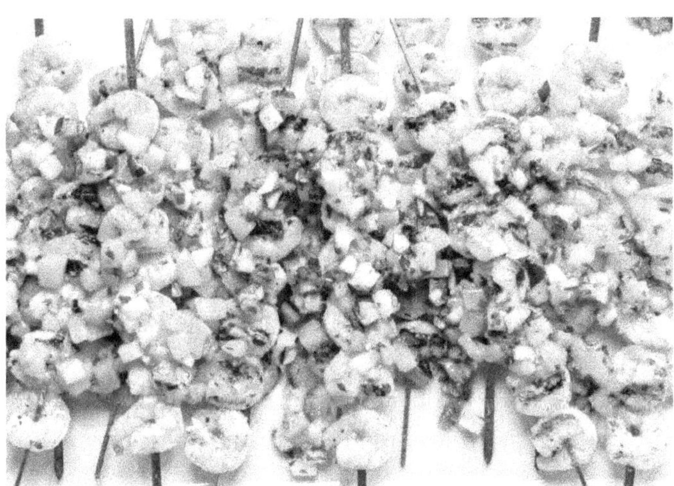

Shrimp and Pineapple Skewers
Ingredients:
- 12 large shrimp, peeled and deveined

- 1 cup pineapple chunks
- 1/4 cup coconut oil
- 2 tbsp lime juice
- 1 tsp ground cumin
- Salt and pepper to taste

Spicy Mango Sauce
Ingredients:
- 2 ripe mangos, diced
- 1/4 cup coconut cream
- 1 tbsp honey
- 1 tsp grated ginger
- 1/4 tsp cayenne pepper

Cauliflower Rice
Ingredients:
- 1 head of cauliflower, grated
- 2 tbsp coconut oil
- Salt and pepper to taste

Instructions:
1. Grill the shrimp and pineapple skewers with coconut oil, lime juice, and cumin.
2. Blend the mango sauce ingredients until smooth.
3. Sauté the cauliflower rice with coconut oil and season with salt and pepper.
4. Serve the shrimp and pineapple skewers with spicy mango sauce and cauliflower rice.

Satisfying Dinner Recipes

1. Grilled Chicken and Vegetable Skewers with Quinoa

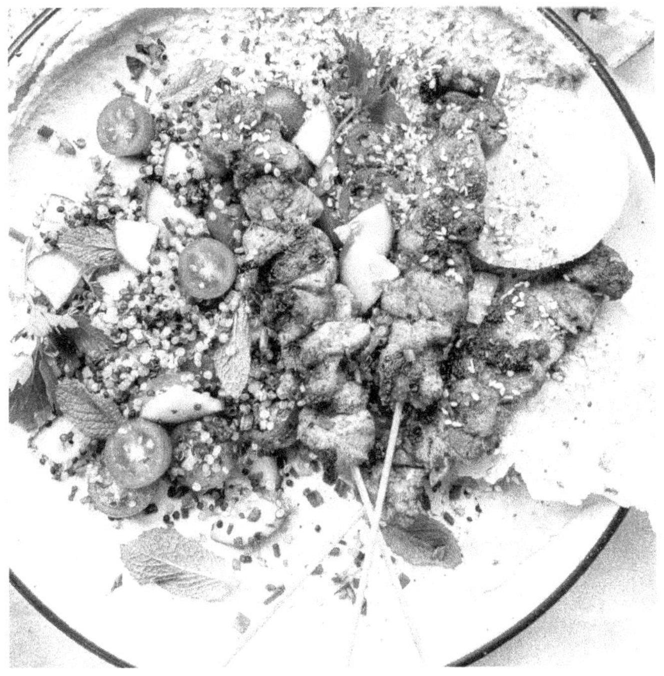

Ingredients:
- 4 boneless, skinless chicken breasts, cut into
1-inch pieces
- 1 cup mixed vegetables, such as cherry tomatoes,
bell peppers, onions, and mushrooms
- 1/2 cup quinoa
- 2 cups water
- 2 tablespoons olive oil

- 1 tablespoon lemon juice
- 1 clove garlic, minced
- Salt and pepper to taste

Instructions:
1. Preheat the grill to medium-high heat.
2. Thread chicken and vegetables onto skewers.
3. In a small bowl, whisk together olive oil, lemon juice, garlic, salt, and pepper. Brush the mixture onto the skewers.
4. Grill for 10-12 minutes, or until chicken is cooked through.
5. Cook quinoa according to package instructions.
6. Serve skewers over quinoa.

Tips:
- Use any color bell pepper you like!
- Add a sprinkle of paprika for extra flavor.
- Make ahead: Prepare quinoa and skewers ahead of time.

2. Baked Salmon with Sweet Potato and Green Beans

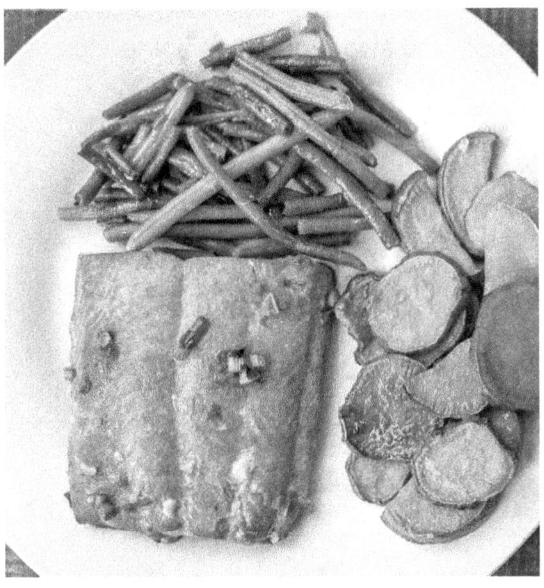

Ingredients:
- 4 salmon filets (6 ounces each)
- 2 large sweet potatoes, peeled and cubed
- 2 cups green beans, trimmed
- 2 tablespoons olive oil
- 1 tablespoon lemon juice
- 1 clove garlic, minced
- Salt and pepper to taste

Instructions:
1. Preheat the oven to 400°F.
2. Line a baking sheet with parchment paper.
3. Place salmon filets on the baking sheet.

4. Toss sweet potatoes and green beans with olive oil, lemon juice, garlic, salt, and pepper. Spread on the baking sheet with the salmon.
5. Bake for 12-15 minutes, or until salmon is cooked through and sweet potatoes are tender.

Tips:
- Use any color sweet potato you like!
- Add a sprinkle of paprika for extra flavor.
- Make ahead: Prepare sweet potatoes and green beans ahead of time.

3. Lentil And Vegetable Stew With Brown Rice

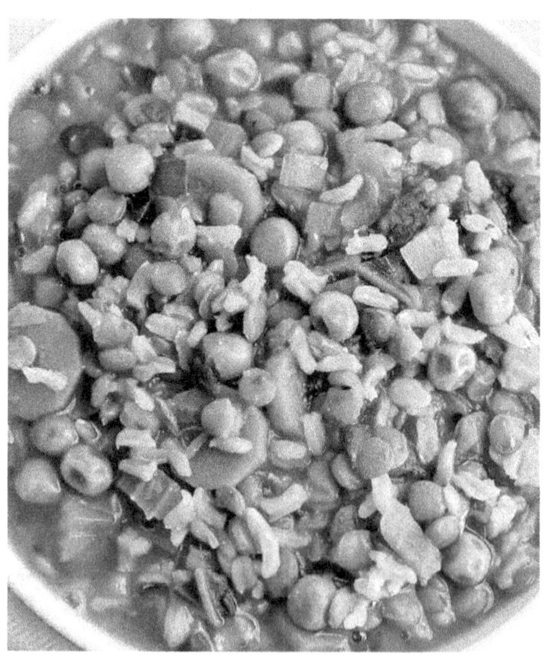

Ingredients:

- 1 cup brown rice
- 2 cups water
- 1 cup red or green lentils, rinsed and drained
- 2 cups vegetable broth
- 1 onion, chopped
- 2 cloves garlic, minced
- 1 carrot, chopped
- 1 celery stalk, chopped
- 1 can diced tomatoes
- 1 teaspoon dried thyme
- Salt and pepper to taste

Instructions:

1. Cook brown rice according to package instructions.
2. In a pot, sauté onion, garlic, carrot, and celery until tender.
3. Add lentils, vegetable broth, diced tomatoes, thyme, salt, and pepper. Simmer for 20-25 minutes, or until lentils are tender.
4. Serve stew over brown rice.

Tips:

- Use any color lentils you like!
- Add a sprinkle of paprika for extra flavor.
- Make ahead: Prepare stew and rice ahead of time.

4. Grilled Turkey Burgers With Avocado And Sweet Potato Fries

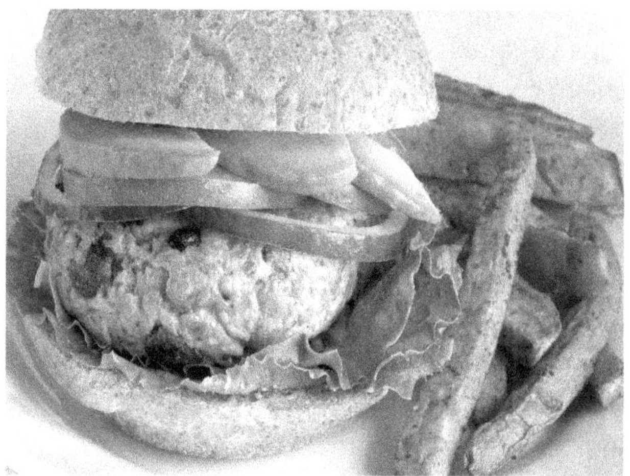

Ingredients:
- 4 turkey burgers (made with lean ground turkey)
- 2 ripe avocados, sliced
- 2 large sweet potatoes, peeled and cut into fries
- 1/2 cup olive oil
- Salt and pepper to taste

Instructions:
1. Preheat the grill to medium-high heat.
2. Grill turkey burgers for 5-6 minutes per side, or until cooked through.
3. Toss sweet potato fries with olive oil, salt, and pepper. Grill or bake until crispy.
4. Serve burgers on a whole-grain bun with avocado slices and sweet potato fries.

Tips:
- Use whole-grain buns for extra fiber!
- Add a sprinkle of paprika for extra flavor.
- Make ahead: Prepare sweet potato fries ahead of time.

5. Roasted Vegetables And Black Bean Chili With Quinoa

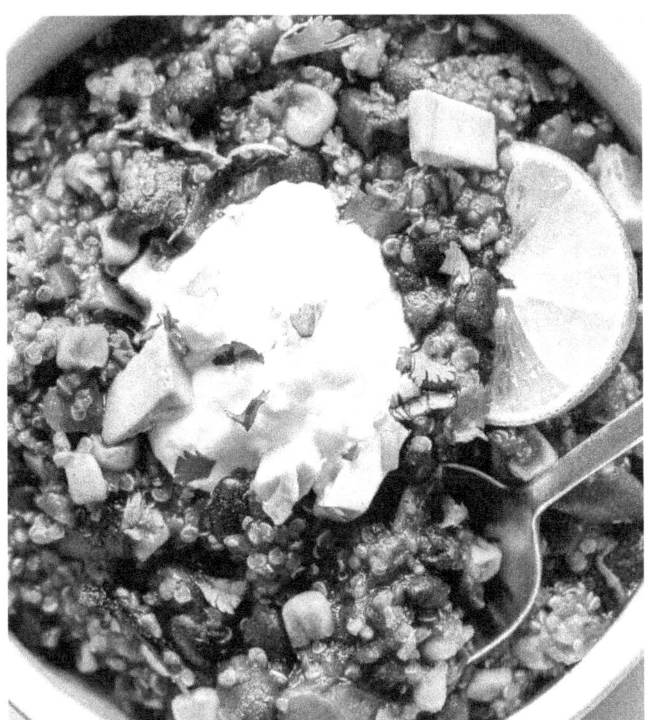

Ingredients:
- 1 cup quinoa
- 2 cups water
- 1 can black beans, drained and rinsed

- 2 cups mixed roasted vegetables (such as sweet potatoes, carrots, and onions)
- 1 can diced tomatoes
- 1 teaspoon cumin
- 1 teaspoon chili powder
- Salt and pepper to taste

Instructions:

1. Cook quinoa according to package instructions.
2. In a pot, combine black beans, roasted vegetables, diced tomatoes, cumin, chili powder, salt, and pepper. Simmer for 10-15 minutes.
3. Serve chili over quinoa.

Tips:

- Use any color bell pepper you like!
- Add a sprinkle of paprika for extra flavor.
- Make ahead: Prepare chili and quinoa ahead of time.

6. Grilled Shrimp And Vegetable Stir-Fry With Brown Rice

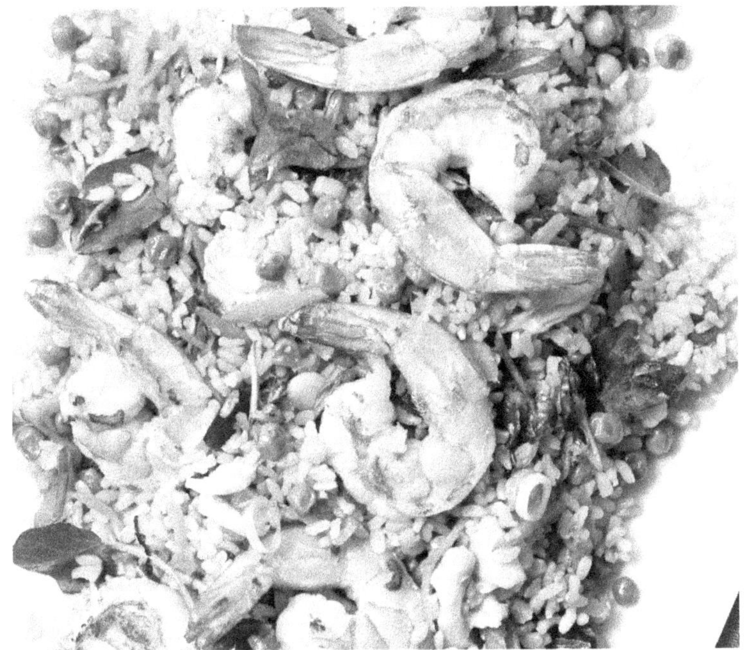

Ingredients:

- 1 cup brown rice
- 2 cups water
- 1 pound large shrimp, peeled and deveined
- 2 cups mixed vegetables (such as broccoli, bell peppers, and onions)
- 2 tablespoons olive oil
- 1 tablespoon soy sauce
- 1 tablespoon honey
- Salt and pepper to taste

Instructions:

1. Cook brown rice according to package instructions.
2. Grill shrimp until pink and cooked through.
3. In a separate pan, stir-fry vegetables with olive oil, soy sauce, and honey until tender.
4. Serve shrimp and vegetables over brown rice.

Tips:
- Use any color of bell pepper you like
- Add a sprinkle of paprika for extra flavor.
- Make ahead: Prepare rice and stir-fry ahead of time.

7. Spinach And Feta Stuffed Chicken Breast With Roasted Asparagus

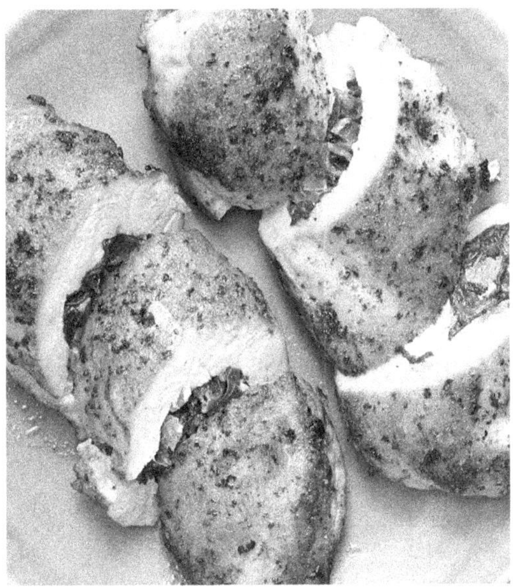

Ingredients:
- 4 boneless, skinless chicken breasts
- 1 package frozen chopped spinach, thawed and drained
- 1/2 cup crumbled feta cheese
- 2 cloves garlic, minced
- 1 pound fresh asparagus, trimmed
- 2 tablespoons olive oil
- Salt and pepper to taste

Instructions:
1. Preheat the oven to 375°F.

2. In a bowl, mix spinach, feta cheese, and garlic.
3. Stuff each chicken breast with the spinach mixture and bake for 20-25 minutes or until cooked through.
4. Toss asparagus with olive oil, salt, and pepper. Roast in the oven for 10-12 minutes or until tender.

Tips:
- Use fresh spinach if available!
- Add a sprinkle of paprika for extra flavor.
- Make ahead: Prepare spinach mixture and asparagus ahead of time.

8. Vegetables And Bean Curry With Brown Rice And Naan Bread

Ingredients:
- 1 cup brown rice
- 2 cups water
- 1 can black beans, drained and rinsed
- 2 cups mixed vegetables (such as carrots, potatoes, and peas)
- 2 tablespoons curry powder
- 1 teaspoon turmeric
- 1/2 teaspoon cumin
- 1/4 teaspoon cayenne pepper (optional)
- 1 can coconut milk
- Salt and pepper to taste
- 4 naan breads

Instructions:

1. Cook brown rice according to package instructions.
2. In a pot, combine black beans, mixed vegetables, curry powder, turmeric, cumin, cayenne pepper (if using), and coconut milk. Simmer for 10-15 minutes.
3. Serve curry over brown rice with naan bread on the side.

Tips:

- Use any color bell pepper you like!
- Add a sprinkle of paprika for extra flavor.
- Make ahead: Prepare curry and rice ahead of time.

9. Grilled Chicken And Quinoa Bowl With Roasted Vegetables

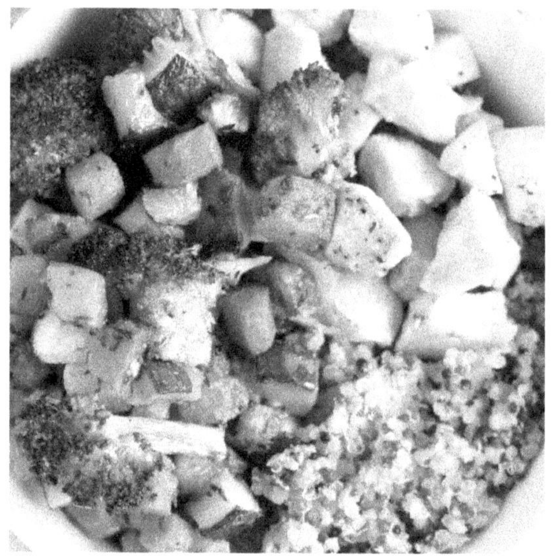

Ingredients:
- 1 cup quinoa
- 2 cups water
- 4 boneless, skinless chicken breasts
- 2 cups mixed vegetables (such as broccoli, carrots, and bell peppers)
- 2 tablespoons olive oil
- 1 tablespoon lemon juice
- Salt and pepper to taste

Instructions:
1. Cook quinoa according to package instructions.
2. Grill chicken breasts until cooked through.

3. Toss vegetables with olive oil, lemon juice, salt, and pepper. Roast in the oven until tender.
4. Serve grilled chicken on top of quinoa with roasted vegetables.

Tips:
- Use any color bell pepper you like!
- Add a sprinkle of paprika for extra flavor.
- Make ahead: Prepare quinoa and roast vegetables ahead of time.

10. Baked Cod With Lemon And Herbs With Roasted Carrots And Brussels Sprouts

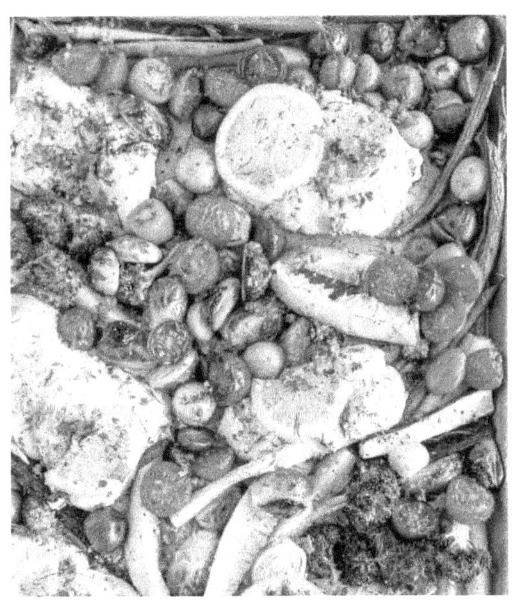

Ingredients:
- 4 cod filets (6 ounces each)
- 2 lemons, sliced
- 1/4 cup olive oil
- 4 sprigs fresh rosemary
- 4 sprigs fresh thyme
- Salt and pepper to taste
- 2 large carrots, peeled and chopped
- 1 pound Brussels sprouts, trimmed

Instructions:
1. Preheat the oven to 400°F.
2. Line a baking sheet with parchment paper.
3. Place cod filets on the baking sheet.
4. Drizzle with olive oil and top with lemon slices, rosemary, and thyme.
5. Season with salt and pepper.
6. Roast in the oven for 12-15 minutes or until cooked through.
7. Toss carrots and Brussels sprouts with olive oil, salt, and pepper. Roast in the oven for 20-25 minutes or until tender.

Tips:
- Use fresh herbs for the best flavor!
- Add a sprinkle of paprika for extra flavor.
- Make ahead: Prepare cod and vegetables ahead of time.

11. Chickpea And Spinach Curry With Brown Rice

Ingredients:
- 1 cup brown rice
- 2 cups water
- 1 can chickpeas, drained and rinsed
- 2 cups fresh spinach leaves
- 2 tablespoons curry powder
- 1 teaspoon ground cumin
- 1/2 teaspoon turmeric
- 1/4 teaspoon cayenne pepper (optional)
- 1 can coconut milk
- Salt and pepper to taste

Instructions:
1. Cook brown rice according to package instructions.
2. In a pot, combine chickpeas, spinach, curry powder, cumin, turmeric, cayenne pepper (if using), and coconut milk. Simmer for 10-15 minutes or until spinach is wilted.
3. Serve curry over brown rice.

Tips:
- Use fresh spinach for the best flavor!
- Add a sprinkle of paprika for extra flavor.
- Make ahead: Prepare curry and rice ahead of time.

12. Lentil Soup With Whole Grain Bread

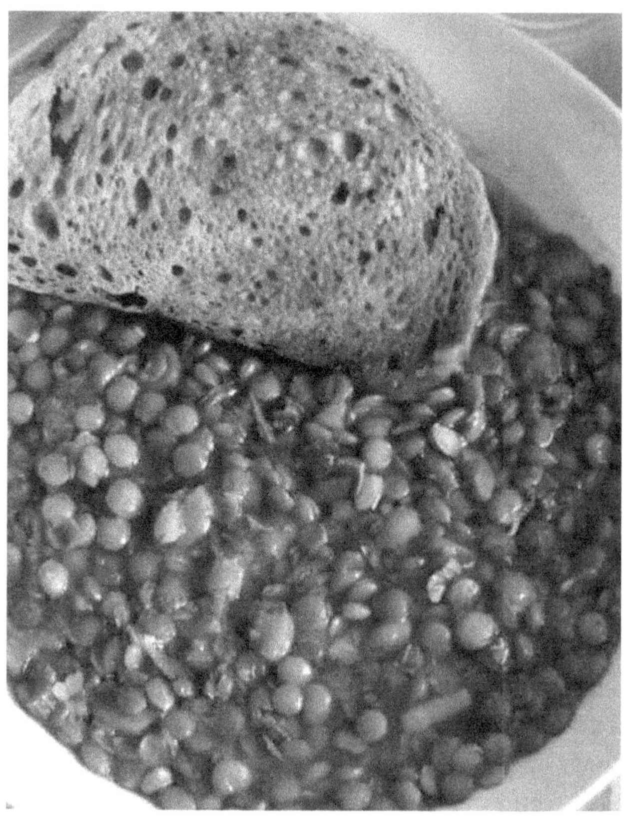

Ingredients:

- 1 cup dried green or brown lentils, rinsed and drained
- 4 cups vegetable broth
- 1 onion, chopped
- 2 cloves garlic, minced
- 1 carrot, chopped
- 1 celery stalk, chopped

- 1 can diced tomatoes
- 1 teaspoon dried thyme
- Salt and pepper to taste
- 2 slices whole grain bread

Instructions:
1. In a pot, combine lentils, vegetable broth, onion, garlic, carrot, celery, diced tomatoes, and thyme.
2. Bring to a boil, then reduce heat and simmer for 30-40 minutes or until lentils are tender.
3. Serve with whole grain bread.

Tips:
- Use red or yellow lentils for a different flavor.
- Add a sprinkle of paprika for extra flavor.
- Make ahead: Prepare soup ahead of time.

13. Beef And Vegetable Stir-Fry With Brown Rice

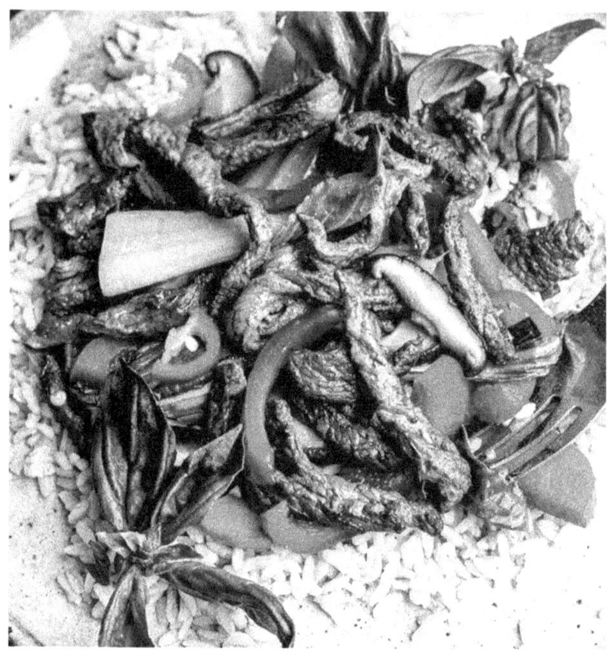

Beef and Vegetable Stir-Fry
Ingredients:
- 4 oz beef strips (sirloin or ribeye, sliced)
- 2 cups mixed vegetables (broccoli, carrots, bell peppers, snow peas)
- 2 cloves garlic, minced
- 1 tbsp coconut oil
- 1 tsp soy sauce (low-sodium)
- 1 tsp oyster sauce (optional)
- Salt and pepper, to taste

Brown Rice

Ingredients:
- 1 cup brown rice
- 2 cups water
- Salt, to taste

Instructions:
1. Cook brown rice according to package instructions.
2. In a large skillet or wok, heat coconut oil over medium-high heat.
3. Add beef and cook until browned, about 3-4 minutes. Remove from the skillet.
4. Add garlic, mixed vegetables, soy sauce, and oyster sauce (if using). Cook until vegetables are tender-crisp.
5. Return beef to the skillet and stir to combine.
6. Serve beef and vegetable stir-fry over brown rice.

14. Baked Chicken Thighs With Roasted Brussels Sprouts And Sweet Potatoes

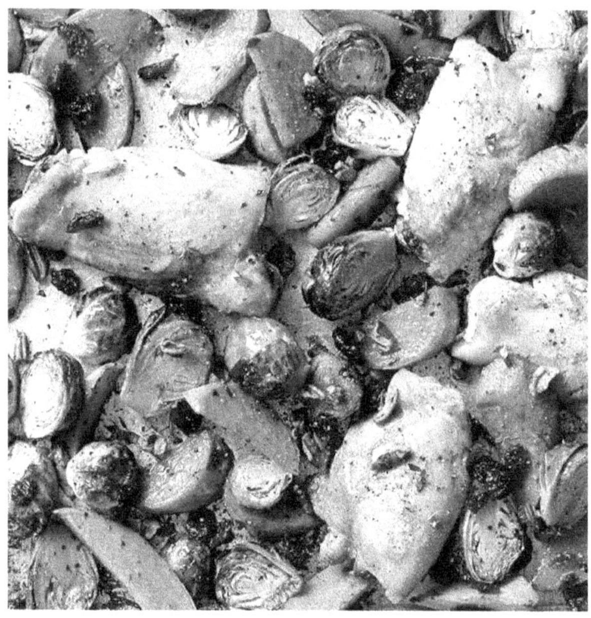

Baked Chicken Thighs
Ingredients:
- 4 bone-in, skin-on chicken thighs
- 2 tbsp olive oil
- 1 tsp salt
- 1 tsp pepper
- 1 tsp garlic powder
- 1 tsp paprika

Roasted Brussels Sprouts
Ingredients:

- 1 pound Brussels sprouts, trimmed and halved
- 2 tbsp olive oil
- Salt and pepper, to taste

Roasted Sweet Potatoes
Ingredients:
- 2 large sweet potatoes, peeled and cubed
- 2 tbsp olive oil
- Salt and pepper, to taste

Instructions:
1. Preheat the oven to 400°F (200°C).
2. In a large bowl, mix olive oil, salt, pepper, garlic powder, and paprika. Add chicken thighs and toss to coat.
3. Spread Brussels sprouts on a baking sheet, drizzle with olive oil, and season with salt and pepper.
4. Spread sweet potatoes on a separate baking sheet, drizzle with olive oil, and season with salt and pepper.
5. Bake chicken thighs for 25-30 minutes or until cooked through.
6. Roast Brussels sprouts and sweet potatoes for 20-25 minutes or until tender.
7. Serve baked chicken thighs with roasted Brussels sprouts and sweet potatoes.

15. Grilled Pork Chops With Roasted Vegetables And Sweet Potatoes

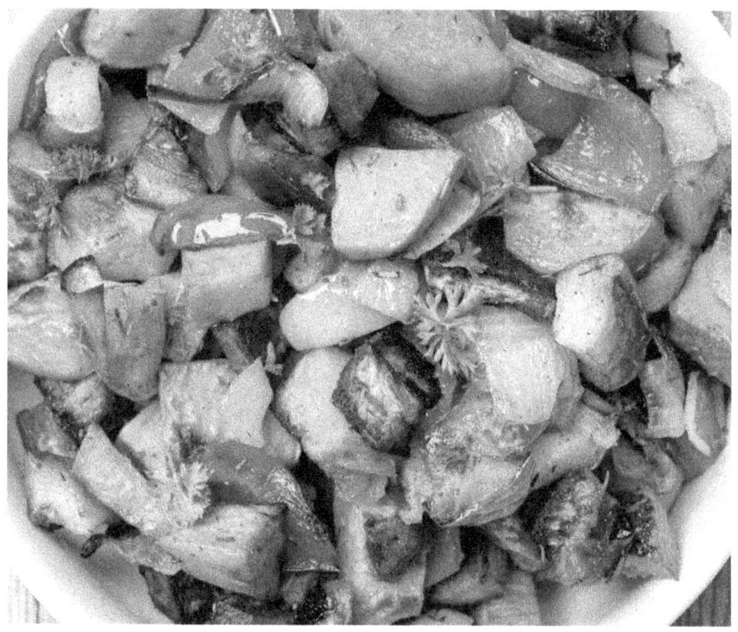

Grilled Pork Chops
Ingredients:

- 4 pork chops (6 oz each, boneless)
- 2 tbsp olive oil
- 1 tsp salt
- 1 tsp pepper
- 1 tsp paprika
- 1 tsp garlic powder

Roasted Vegetables
Ingredients:

- 1 large red bell pepper, seeded and sliced
- 1 large yellow bell pepper, seeded and sliced
- 2 large zucchinis, sliced
- 2 large red onions, sliced
- 3 cloves garlic, minced
- 2 tbsp olive oil
- Salt and pepper, to taste

Sweet Potatoes
Ingredients:
- 2 large sweet potatoes, peeled and cubed
- 2 tbsp olive oil
- Salt and pepper, to taste

Instructions:
1. Preheat the grill to medium-high heat.
2. In a small bowl, mix olive oil, salt, pepper, paprika, and garlic powder. Rub the spice blend on both sides of the pork chops.
3. Grill pork chops for 5-6 minutes per side or until cooked through. Let rest for 5 minutes before slicing.
4. Toss vegetables with olive oil, salt, and pepper on a baking sheet. Roast in the oven at 425°F (220°C) for 25-30 minutes or until tender.
5. Toss sweet potatoes with olive oil, salt, and pepper on a separate baking sheet. Roast in the oven at 425°F (220°C) for 20-25 minutes or until tender.
6. Serve sliced pork chops with roasted vegetables and sweet potatoes

Chapter Four

Hearty Soups And Stews

1. Vegetable Broth With Kale And Quinoa

Ingredients:
- 2 cups mixed vegetables (such as carrots, celery, onions, spinach, zucchini, bell peppers, and mushrooms)
- 4 cups water
- 2 cups kale, stems removed and chopped
- 1 cup quinoa, rinsed and drained
- 2 tablespoons olive oil
- Salt and pepper, to taste
- Optional: 1 teaspoon dried thyme, 1/2 teaspoon garlic powder

Instructions:
1. In a large pot, sauté the mixed vegetables in olive oil until tender.
2. Add water, kale, quinoa, thyme (if using), and garlic powder (if using).
3. Bring to a boil, then reduce heat and simmer for 20-25 minutes or until quinoa is tender.
4. Season with salt and pepper to taste.
5. Serve hot and enjoy!

This recipe makes about 6 servings. You can store leftovers in the refrigerator for up to 3 days or freeze for up to 2 months.

Note: You can customize the recipe by using different vegetables or adding protein sources like chickpeas or tofu.

2. Lentil Soup With Spinach And Feta

Ingredients:
- 1 cup dried green or brown lentils, rinsed and drained
- 4 cups water
- 1 onion, chopped
- 2 cloves garlic, minced
- 1 carrot, chopped
- 1 celery stalk, chopped
- 1 can (14.5 oz) diced tomatoes
- 2 cups fresh spinach leaves
- 1/2 cup crumbled feta cheese
- 1 teaspoon dried thyme
- Salt and pepper, to taste
- Optional: 1/4 teaspoon red pepper flakes (for some heat)

Instructions:
1. In a large pot, sauté the onion, garlic, carrot, and celery in olive oil until tender.

2. Add lentils, water, diced tomatoes, thyme, and red pepper flakes (if using).
3. Bring to a boil, then reduce heat and simmer for 30-35 minutes or until lentils are tender.
4. Stir in spinach and cook until wilted.
5. Season with salt and pepper to taste.
6. Serve hot, topped with crumbled feta cheese.

Tip:
Use a pressure cooker to reduce cooking time to 15-20 minutes. Also, add a squeeze of lemon juice for extra flavor.

3. Roasted Butternut Squash And Apple Soup

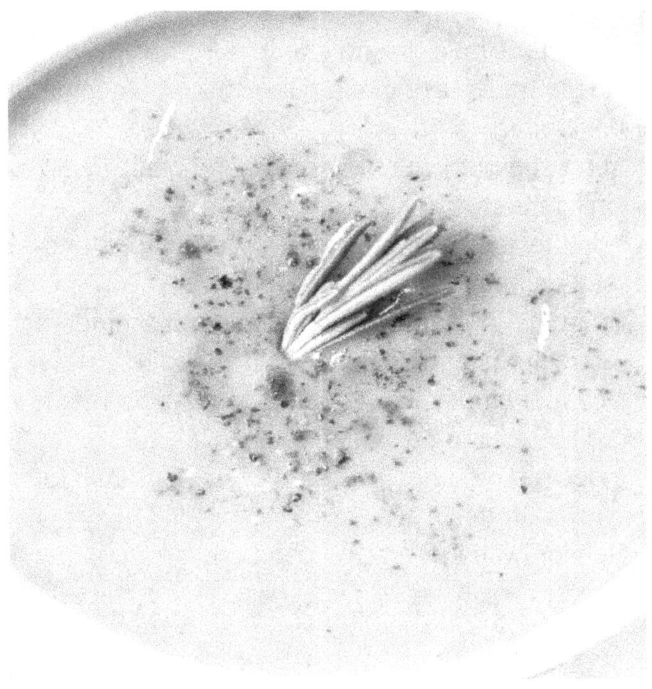

Ingredients:
- 1 large butternut squash (about 2 lbs)
- 2 apples, peeled and chopped
- 2 tablespoons olive oil
- 1 onion, chopped
- 3 cloves garlic, minced
- 4 cups vegetable broth
- 1/2 cup heavy cream or half-and-half (optional)
- Salt and pepper, to taste
- Optional: nutmeg, cinnamon, or paprika for added spice

Instructions:
1. Preheat the oven to 400°F (200°C).
2. Cut the squash in half lengthwise and scoop out seeds. Place on a baking sheet, cut side up.
3. Roast the squash in the oven for 45-50 minutes, or until tender.
4. In a large pot, sauté the onion and garlic in olive oil until tender.
5. Add the chopped apples, vegetable broth, and roasted squash flesh to the pot.
6. Bring to a boil, then reduce heat and simmer for 15-20 minutes or until the soup is smooth.
7. Use an immersion blender or regular blender to puree the soup until smooth.
8. If desired, add heavy cream or half-and-half for a creamy texture.
9. Season with salt, pepper, and any desired spices.
10. Serve hot and enjoy!

Tip:
Use pre-cut butternut squash or apple chunks to save time on prep work. Also, add a splash of apple cider vinegar for a tangy flavor boost.

4. Chickpea And Spinach Curry Soup

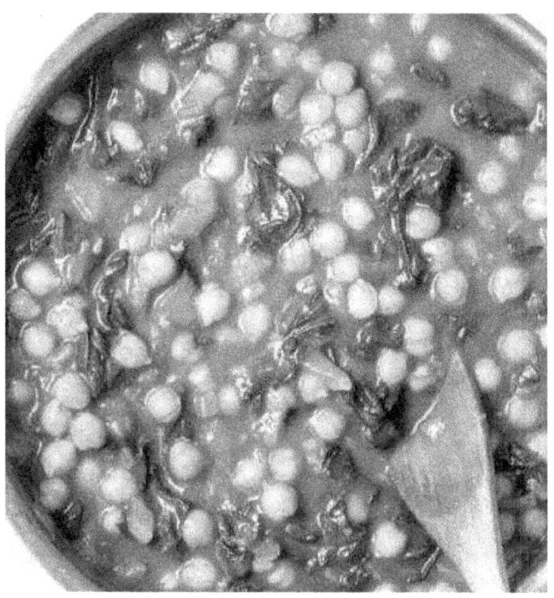

Ingredients:
- 1 can (14.5 oz) chickpeas, drained and rinsed
- 2 cups fresh spinach leaves
- 1 onion, chopped
- 2 cloves garlic, minced
- 1 tablespoon curry powder
- 1 teaspoon ground cumin
- 1/2 teaspoon turmeric
- 1/2 teaspoon cayenne pepper (optional)
- 1 can (14 oz) coconut milk
- 4 cups vegetable broth
- Salt and pepper, to taste
- Fresh cilantro leaves for garnish (optional)

Instructions:

1. In a large pot, sauté the onion and garlic in olive oil until tender.
2. Add the curry powder, cumin, turmeric, and cayenne pepper (if using) and cook for 1-2 minutes.
3. Stir in the chickpeas, spinach, coconut milk, and vegetable broth.
4. Bring to a boil, then reduce heat and simmer for 15-20 minutes or until the spinach is wilted.
5. Season with salt and pepper to taste.
6. Serve hot, garnished with fresh cilantro leaves if desired.

Tip:

Use a pressure cooker to reduce cooking time to 5-7 minutes. Also, add a squeeze of fresh lime juice for extra brightness.

5. Creamy Tomato And Spinach Soup With Greek Yogurt

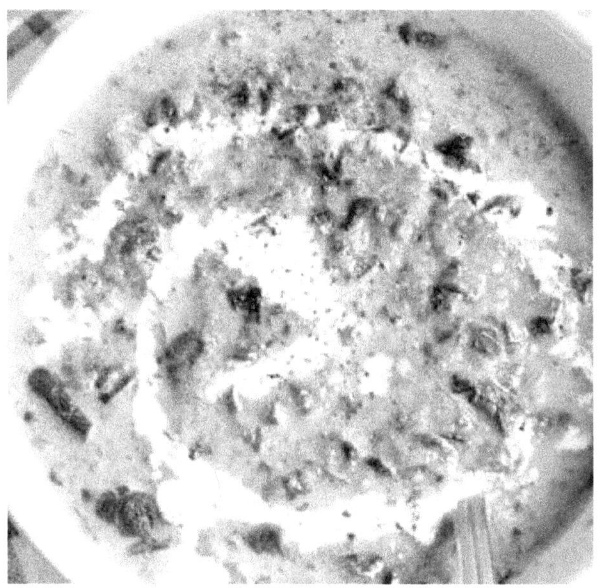

Ingredients:
- 2 tablespoons olive oil
- 1 onion, chopped
- 3 cloves garlic, minced
- 2 cups chopped fresh tomatoes (or 1 can diced tomatoes)
- 2 cups vegetable broth
- 1 cup fresh spinach leaves
- 1/2 cup Greek yogurt
- 1 teaspoon dried basil
- Salt and pepper, to taste
- Optional: 1/4 teaspoon red pepper flakes (for some heat)

Instructions:

1. In a large pot, sauté the onion and garlic in olive oil until tender.
2. Add the chopped tomatoes, vegetable broth, and basil. Bring to a boil, then reduce heat and simmer for 15-20 minutes.
3. Stir in the fresh spinach leaves and cook until wilted.
4. Use an immersion blender or regular blender to puree the soup until smooth.
5. Return the soup to the pot and add the Greek yogurt. Stir over low heat until the yogurt is fully incorporated and the soup is heated through.
6. Season with salt, pepper, and red pepper flakes (if using).
7. Serve hot and enjoy.

Tip:

Use fresh tomatoes when in season, or high-quality canned tomatoes otherwise. Also, add some grated Parmesan cheese for an extra burst of flavor.

6. Black Bean And Sweet Potato Stew With Quinoa

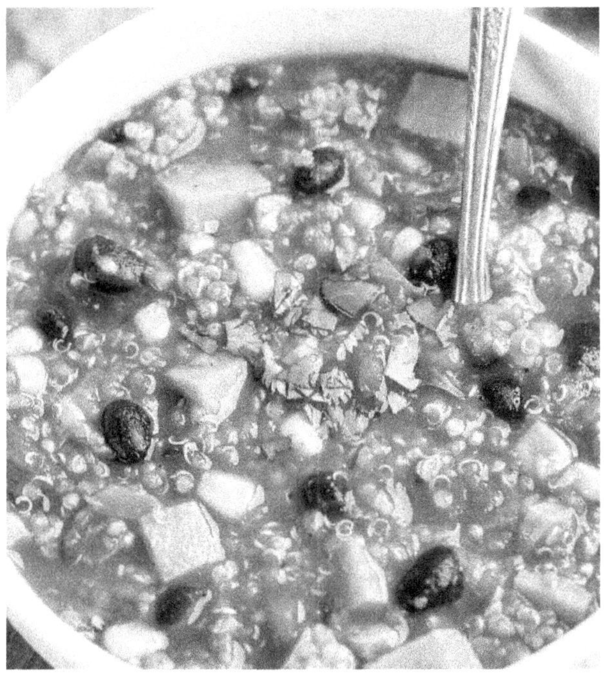

Ingredients:
- 1 medium sweet potato, peeled and chopped
- 1 can (15 oz) black beans, drained and rinsed
- 1 onion, chopped
- 2 cloves garlic, minced
- 1 red bell pepper, chopped
- 2 cups vegetable broth
- 1 cup quinoa, rinsed and drained
- 1 teaspoon cumin
- 1 teaspoon smoked paprika (optional)
- Salt and pepper, to taste

- Fresh cilantro leaves for garnish (optional)

Instructions:
1. In a large pot, sauté the onion, garlic, and red bell pepper in olive oil until tender.
2. Add the chopped sweet potato, black beans, vegetable broth, quinoa, cumin, and smoked paprika (if using).
3. Bring to a boil, then reduce heat and simmer for 20-25 minutes or until the sweet potato is tender and the quinoa is cooked.
4. Season with salt and pepper to taste.
5. Serve hot, garnished with fresh cilantro leaves if desired.

Tip:
Use pre-cooked quinoa to save time, and add some diced tomatoes for extra flavor.

7. Lentil And Vegetables Stew With Brown Rice

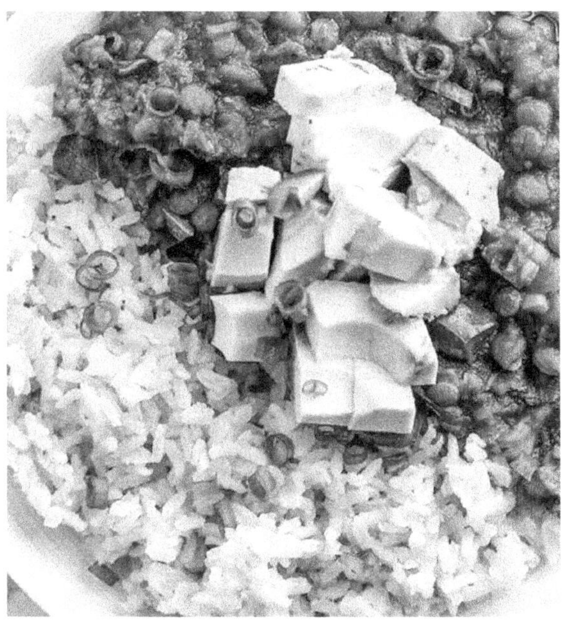

Ingredients:
- 1 cup dried green or brown lentils, rinsed and drained
- 2 cups water
- 1 onion, chopped
- 2 cloves garlic, minced
- 2 carrots, chopped
- 2 potatoes, chopped
- 1 cup mixed vegetables (such as zucchini, bell peppers, and tomatoes)
- 2 cups vegetable broth
- 1 cup cooked brown rice
- 1 teaspoon dried thyme

- Salt and pepper, to taste
- Optional: 1/4 teaspoon cayenne pepper (for some
heat)

Instructions:
1. In a large pot, sauté the onion, garlic, carrots,
and potatoes in olive oil until tender.
2. Add the lentils, water, mixed vegetables,
vegetable broth, thyme, and cayenne pepper (if
using).
3. Bring to a boil, then reduce heat and simmer for
30-35 minutes or until the lentils are tender.
4. Serve the stew over cooked brown rice.

Tip:
Use red or yellow lentils for a softer texture, and
add some chopped fresh spinach for extra nutrition.

8. Chicken And Vegetables Stew With Kale And Quinoa

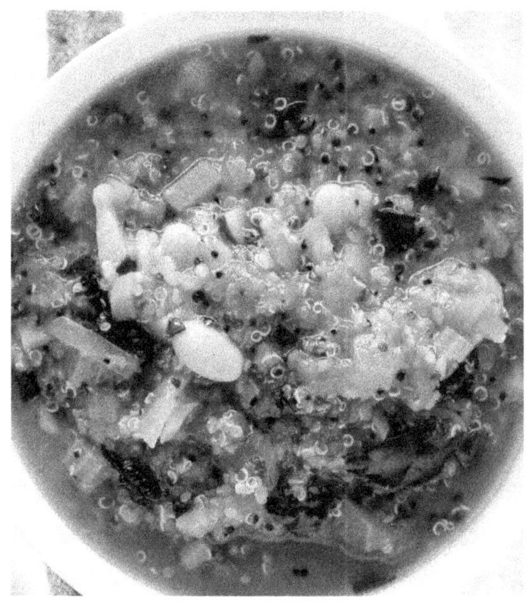

Ingredients:
- 1 pound boneless, skinless chicken breast or thighs, cut into bite-sized pieces
- 2 cups mixed vegetables (such as carrots, potatoes, and onions)
- 2 cups kale, stems removed and chopped
- 1 cup quinoa, rinsed and drained
- 4 cups chicken broth
- 1 teaspoon dried thyme
- Salt and pepper, to taste
- Optional: 1/4 teaspoon red pepper flakes (for some heat)

Instructions:
1. In a large pot, sauté the chicken and mixed vegetables in olive oil until the chicken is cooked through and the vegetables are tender.
2. Add the chopped kale, quinoa, chicken broth, thyme, and red pepper flakes (if using).
3. Bring to a boil, then reduce heat and simmer for 15-20 minutes or until the quinoa is tender and the kale is wilted.
4. Season with salt and pepper to taste.
5. Serve hot and enjoy.

Tip:
Use pre-cooked chicken or quinoa to save time, and add some diced bell peppers for extra flavor.

9. Vegetables And Bean Stew With Spinach And Feta

Ingredients:
- 1 can (14.5 oz) diced tomatoes
- 1 can (15 oz) kidney beans, drained and rinsed
- 1 onion, chopped
- 2 cloves garlic, minced
- 2 carrots, chopped
- 2 potatoes, chopped
- 1 cup mixed vegetables (such as zucchini, bell peppers, and mushrooms)
- 2 cups vegetable broth
- 1 cup fresh spinach leaves
- 1/2 cup crumbled feta cheese

- 1 teaspoon dried oregano
- Salt and pepper, to taste
- Optional: 1/4 teaspoon red pepper flakes (for some heat)

Instructions:
1. In a large pot, sauté the onion, garlic, carrots, and potatoes in olive oil until tender.
2. Add the diced tomatoes, kidney beans, mixed vegetables, vegetable broth, oregano, and red pepper flakes (if using).
3. Bring to a boil, then reduce heat and simmer for 20-25 minutes or until the vegetables are tender.
4. Stir in the fresh spinach leaves and cook until wilted.
5. Serve hot, topped with crumbled feta cheese.

Tip:
Use canned beans for a quicker cooking time, and add some chopped fresh parsley for extra freshness.

10. Minestrone Soup With Whole Grain Pasta And Kale

Ingredients:
- 1 cup whole grain pasta (such as elbow macaroni or ditalini)
- 2 cups vegetable broth
- 1 can (14.5 oz) diced tomatoes
- 1 cup chopped kale, stems removed

- 1 cup canned kidney beans, drained and rinsed
- 1 cup canned cannellini beans, drained and rinsed
- 1 onion, chopped
- 2 cloves garlic, minced
- 1 carrot, chopped
- 1 celery stalk, chopped
- 1 can (6 oz) tomato paste
- 1 teaspoon dried basil
- 1 teaspoon dried oregano
- Salt and pepper, to taste
- Grated Parmesan cheese, for serving (optional)

Instructions:
1. Cook the whole grain pasta according to package instructions. Drain and set aside.
2. In a large pot, sauté the onion, garlic, carrot, and celery in olive oil until tender.
3. Add the vegetable broth, diced tomatoes, kale, kidney beans, cannellini beans, tomato paste, basil, oregano, salt, and pepper.
4. Bring to a boil, then reduce heat and simmer for 20-25 minutes or until the kale is wilted.
5. Add the cooked pasta to the pot and stir to combine.
6. Serve hot, topped with grated Parmesan cheese if desired.

Tip:
Use a variety of vegetables and beans to make the soup more hearty, and add some red wine vinegar for a tangy flavor boost!

Mouth-Watering Dessert Recipes

1. Berry Chia Seed Pudding

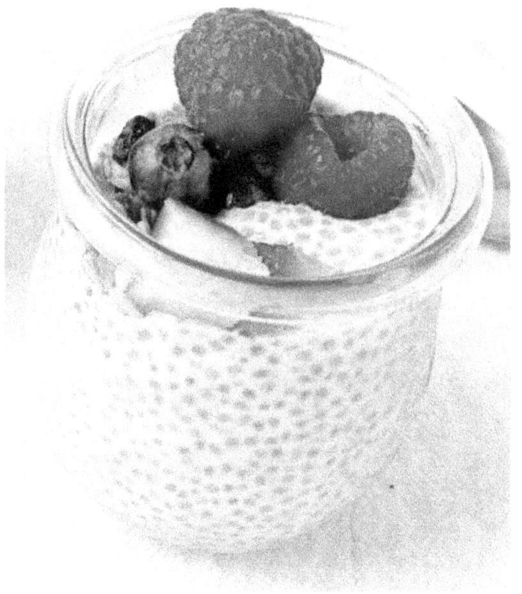

Ingredients:
- 1/2 cup chia seeds
- 1 cup almond milk
- 1/4 cup mixed berries (such as blueberries, raspberries, and blackberries)
- 1 tablespoon honey or stevia
- 1/4 teaspoon vanilla extract

Instructions:

1. In a small bowl, mix together chia seeds, almond milk, and honey or stevia. Whisk well and refrigerate for at least 2 hours or overnight.
2. Add the mixed berries and vanilla extract to the chia seed mixture. Stir well and refrigerate for another 30 minutes.
3. Serve the pudding in individual cups or glasses and enjoy.

Note:
This dessert is not only delicious, but it's also packed with nutrients from the chia seeds, almond milk, and berries. The chia seeds provide a boost of fiber and omega-3 fatty acids, while the berries offer antioxidants and vitamins. This dessert is perfect for women with PCOS who want a sweet treat without compromising their health goals.

2. Dark Chocolate Avocado Mousse

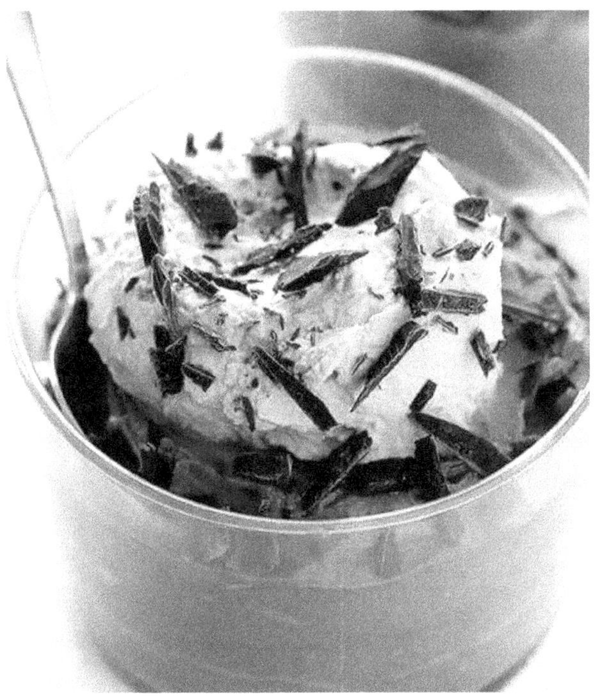

Ingredients:

- 3 ripe avocados
- 1/2 cup dark chocolate chips (at least 85% cocoa)
- 1/4 cup unsweetened almond milk
- 1/4 cup stevia or monk fruit sweetener
- 1/2 teaspoon vanilla extract

Instructions:

1. Peel and pit the avocados and place them in a blender or food processor.

2. Add the cocoa powder, almond milk, sweetener, and vanilla extract to the blender.
3. Blend the mixture until smooth and creamy, stopping to scrape down the sides of the blender as needed.
4. Melt the dark chocolate chips in a double boiler or in the microwave in 30-second increments, stirring between each interval until smooth.
5. Fold the melted chocolate into the avocado mixture until well combined.
6. Spoon the mousse into individual serving cups or glasses and refrigerate for at least 2 hours before serving.

3. Baked Apples With Cinnamon And Oatmeal

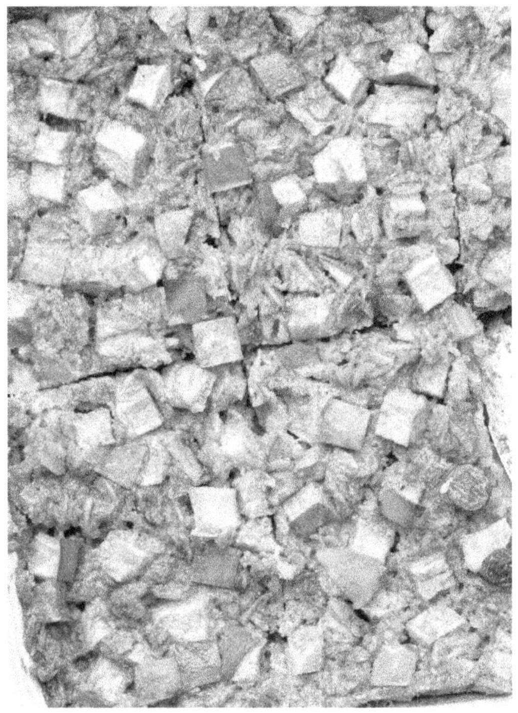

Ingredients:

- 4-6 apples (any variety, cored and halved)
- 1/4 cup rolled oats
- 2 tablespoons cinnamon
- 1/4 teaspoon nutmeg
- 1/4 teaspoon salt
- 1/4 cup unsweetened almond milk
- 1 tablespoon honey or stevia (optional)

Instructions:

1. Preheat the oven to 375°F (190°C).
2. In a bowl, mix together oats, cinnamon, nutmeg, and salt.
3. Add the almond milk and honey or stevia (if using) to the bowl and stir until the mixture is crumbly.
4. Place the apple halves in a baking dish and fill each center with the oat mixture.
5. Bake for 25-30 minutes or until the apples are tender and the topping is golden brown.
6. Serve warm, topped with additional cinnamon if desired.

4. No-Bake Energy Balls

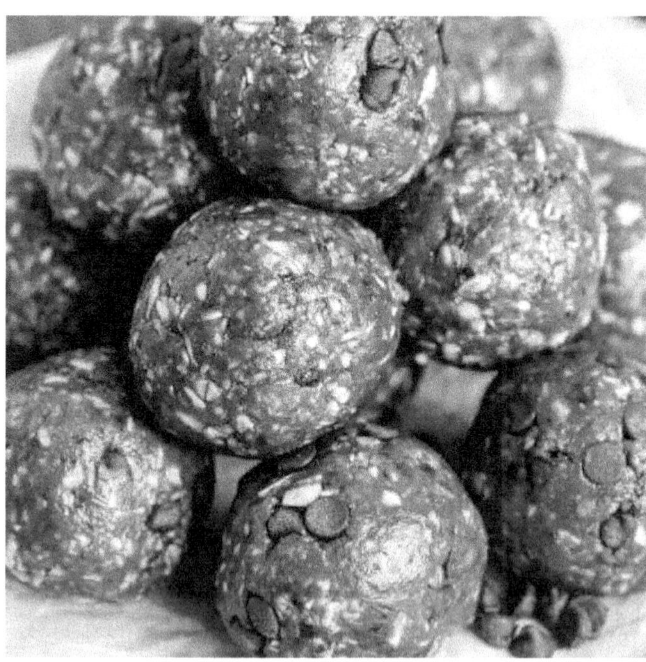

Ingredients:
- 2 cups rolled oats
- 1 cup dried fruit (cranberries, raisins, or cherries)
- 1/2 cup nut butter (peanut butter, almond butter, or cashew butter)
- 1/4 cup honey or stevia
- 1/4 cup chopped nuts (walnuts, almonds, or pecans)
- 1/4 cup chia seeds
- 1/4 cup shredded coconut (optional)

Instructions:
1. In a large bowl, combine oats, dried fruit, and chia seeds.
2. In a small bowl, mix together nut butter and honey or stevia until smooth.
3. Add the nut butter mixture to the oat mixture and stir until everything is well combined.
4. Fold in the chopped nuts and shredded coconut (if using).
5. Use your hands to shape the mixture into small balls, about 1 inch in diameter.
6. Place the energy balls on a baking sheet lined with parchment paper and refrigerate for at least 30 minutes to set.
7. Store in an airtight container in the refrigerator for up to a week.

5. Low-Carb Cheesecake With Fresh Berries

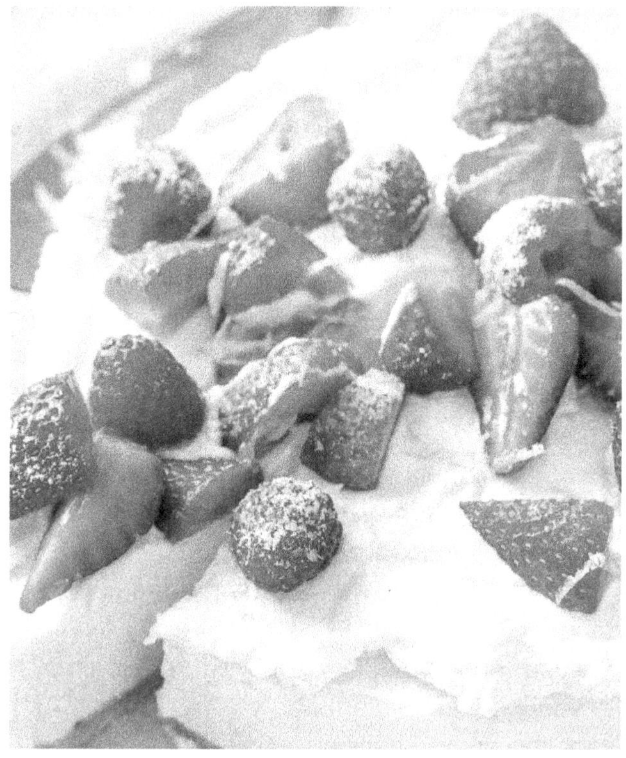

Ingredients:

- 1 1/2 cups almond flour
- 1/2 cup granulated sweetener (such as Swerve or Erythritol)
- 1/4 cup melted coconut oil
- 2 large eggs
- 1/2 cup sour cream
- 1 teaspoon vanilla extract
- 1/2 cup heavy cream

- 1 cup fresh berries (such as strawberries, blueberries, or raspberries)

Instructions:
1. Preheat the oven to 325°F (165°C).
2. Prepare the crust: Mix almond flour, sweetener, and melted coconut oil in a bowl. Press into a 9-inch springform pan.
3. Prepare the filling: Beat eggs, sour cream, and vanilla extract in a separate bowl. Add heavy cream and mix well.
4. Pour filling over the crust and bake for 45-50 minutes or until the edges are set.
5. Let cool completely and top with fresh berries.

6. Chia Seed Coconut Pudding

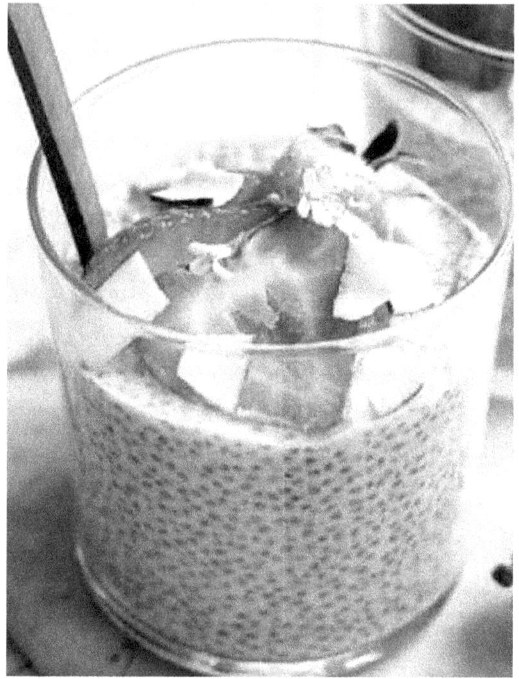

Ingredients:
- 1/2 cup chia seeds
- 1 cup coconut milk
- 1/4 cup unsweetened shredded coconut
- 1/4 cup granulated sweetener (such as Swerve or Erythritol)
- 1/2 teaspoon vanilla extract
- Pinch of salt
- Optional: sliced fruit, nuts, or shredded coconut for topping

Instructions:

1. In a small bowl, mix together chia seeds, coconut milk, unsweetened shredded coconut, sweetener, vanilla extract, and salt.
2. Whisk well and refrigerate for at least 2 hours or overnight.
3. Top with sliced fruit, nuts, or shredded coconut, if desired.
4. Serve chilled and enjoy.

7. Banana "Nice" Cream

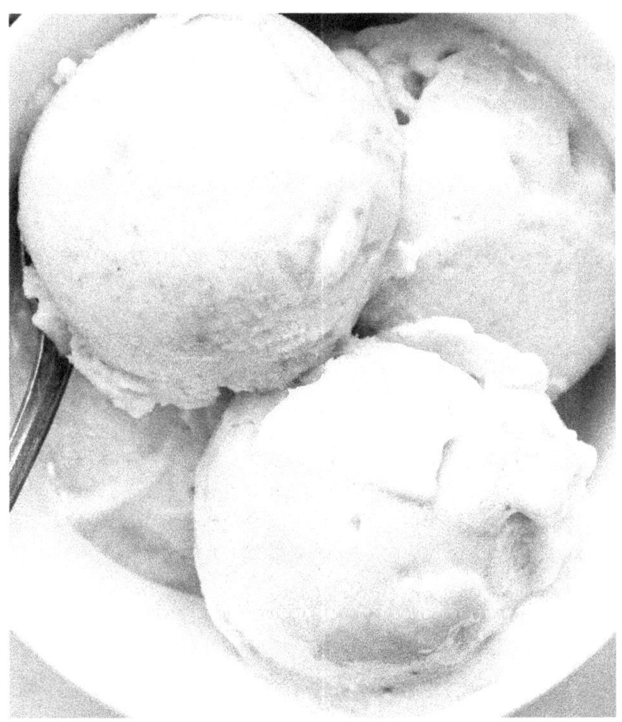

Ingredients:
- 3-4 ripe bananas

- 1/4 cup unsweetened almond milk
- 1/4 cup granulated sweetener (such as Swerve or
Erythritol)
- 1/2 teaspoon vanilla extract
- Pinch of salt
- Optional: mix-ins like cocoa powder, nuts, or fruit

Instructions:
1. Peel the bananas and place them in a
freezer-safe blender or food processor.
2. Add almond milk, sweetener, vanilla extract, and
salt to the blender.
3. Blend the mixture until smooth and creamy,
stopping to scrape down the sides of the blender as
needed.
4. Add mix-ins, if desired, and blend until well
combined.
5. Transfer the "nice" cream to a bowl and serve
immediately.

8. Poached Pears With Cinnamon And Ginger

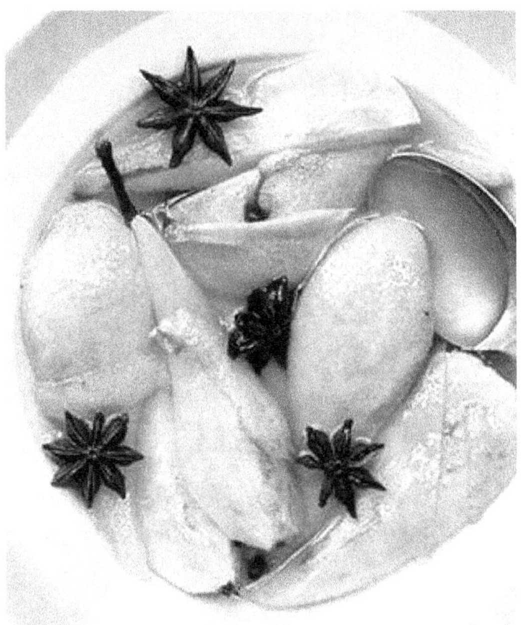

Ingredients:
- 4 ripe pears (such as Bartlett or Anjou)
- 1 cup water
- 1/2 cup granulated sweetener (such as Swerve or Erythritol)
- 1 cinnamon stick
- 1-inch piece of fresh ginger, sliced
- Optional: whipped cream or yogurt for serving

Instructions:
1. Peel, core, and halve the pears.

2. In a large saucepan, combine water, sweetener, cinnamon stick, and ginger slices.

3. Bring the mixture to a boil, then reduce the heat and simmer for 10-12 minutes or until the pears are tender.

4. Remove the pears from the poaching liquid and let them cool.

5. Serve the pears warm or chilled, with whipped cream or yogurt if desired.

9. Low-Sugar Chocolate Chip Cookies

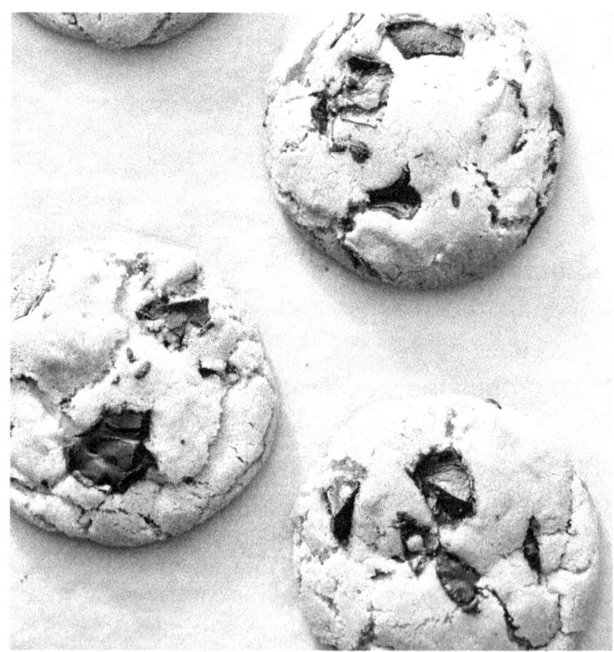

Ingredients:

- 1 cup almond flour
- 1/2 cup coconut sugar
- 1/4 cup granulated sweetener (such as Swerve or Erythritol)
- 1/2 cup unsalted butter, softened
- 2 large eggs
- 1 teaspoon vanilla extract
- 1/2 cup semisweet chocolate chips
- Pinch of salt

Instructions:
1. Preheat the oven to 375°F (190°C). Line a baking sheet with parchment paper.
2. In a medium bowl, whisk together almond flour, coconut sugar, and granulated sweetener.
3. In a separate bowl, whisk together butter, eggs, and vanilla extract.
4. Add the wet ingredients to the dry ingredients and stir until a dough forms. Fold in chocolate chips.
5. Scoop tablespoon-sized balls of dough onto the prepared baking sheet, leaving 2 inches of space between each cookie.
6. Bake for 10-12 minutes or until the edges are lightly golden.
7. Remove from the oven and let cool on the baking sheet for 5 minutes before transferring to a wire rack to cool completely.

10. No-Bake Granola Bars

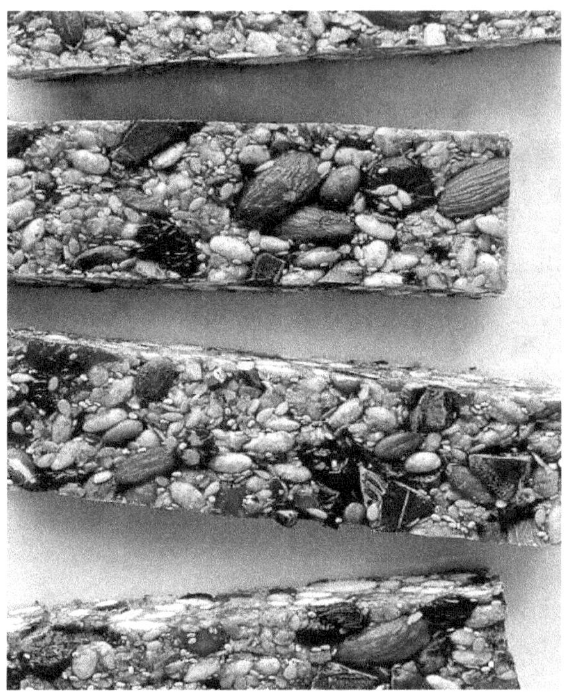

Ingredients:
- 2 cups rolled oats
- 1 cup nut butter (such as peanut butter or almond butter)
- 1/2 cup honey or granulated sweetener (such as Swerve or Erythritol)
- 1/4 cup chopped nuts (such as walnuts or almonds)
- 1/4 cup chia seeds
- 1/4 cup shredded coconut
- Pinch of salt

Instructions:

1. In a large bowl, combine oats, nut butter, and honey or sweetener. Mix until well combined.
2. Fold in chopped nuts, chia seeds, and shredded coconut.
3. Press the mixture into a lined or greased 8x8-inch baking dish.
4. Refrigerate for at least 30 minutes to set.
5. Cut into bars and store in an airtight container in the refrigerator for up to a week.

Note:

These no-bake granola bars are a convenient and healthy dessert option, perfect for snacking on the go. They're packed with fiber, protein, and healthy fats to keep you energized and satisfied. And the best part? No baking required!

Soothing Snack Recipes

1. Fresh Fruit And Nut Butter Wrap

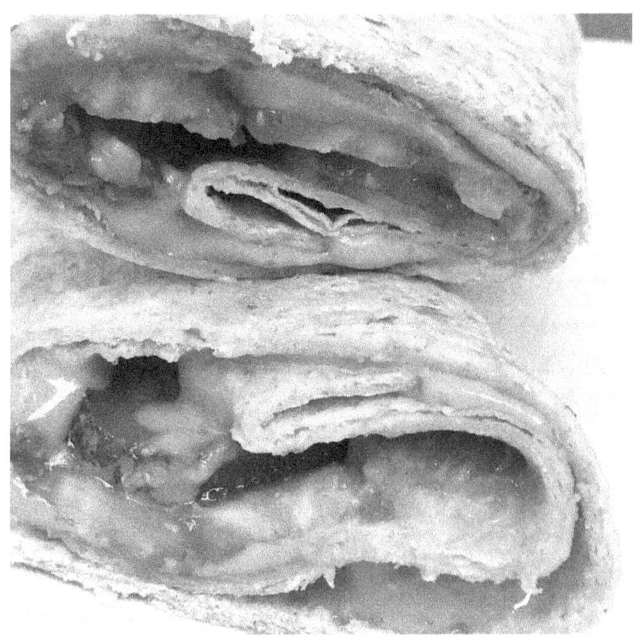

Ingredients:
- 1-2 tablespoons nut butter (such as peanut butter, almond butter, or cashew butter)
- 1-2 cups fresh fruit (such as berries, sliced apples, or sliced bananas)
- 1-2 celery sticks
- Optional: 1/4 teaspoon cinnamon or vanilla extract
- Optional: 1 tablespoon honey or maple syrup (optional)

Instructions:
1. Spread the nut butter on the celery stick, leaving a small border at the top.
2. Top with fresh fruit, leaving a small space between each piece.
3. Sprinkle with cinnamon or vanilla extract, if desired.
4. Drizzle with honey or maple syrup, if desired.
5. Serve and enjoy!

Tips:
- Use a variety of fruits to mix and match your favorite flavors and textures.
- Add a sprinkle of granola or chopped nuts for extra crunch.
- Use a different type of nut butter each time to change up the flavor.
- Consider using a small whole-grain tortilla or wrap instead of celery for a more filling snack.

2. Protein Smoothie

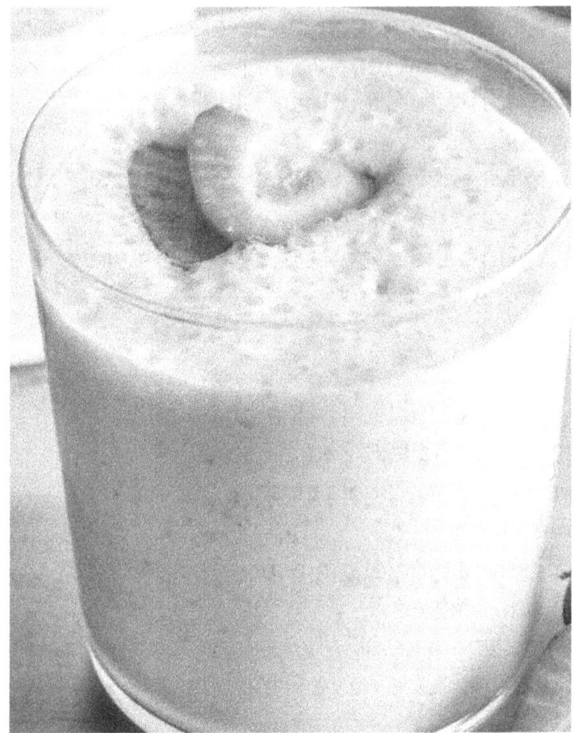

Ingredients:

- 1 scoop vanilla protein powder
- 1/2 cup frozen berries (such as blueberries, strawberries, or raspberries)
- 1/2 cup plain Greek yogurt
- 1/2 cup unsweetened almond milk
- 1 tablespoon chia seeds
- 1 teaspoon honey or stevia (optional)
- Ice cubes (optional)

Instructions:

1. Add all the ingredients to a blender and blend until smooth.
2. Taste and adjust the sweetness by adding more honey or stevia if needed.
3. Add ice cubes if you want a thicker, colder smoothie.
4. Blend again until the ice is crushed and the smoothie is the desired consistency.
5. Pour into a glass and serve immediately.

Tips:
- Use different types of protein powder, such as whey or plant-based options, to change up the flavor and nutritional content.
- Add other fruits, such as bananas or mangoes, to mix and match your favorite flavors.
- Consider adding a handful of spinach or kale for an extra nutritional boost.
- Use coconut milk or another non-dairy milk alternative if you're lactose intolerant or prefer a creamier texture.

3. Roasted Chickpeas

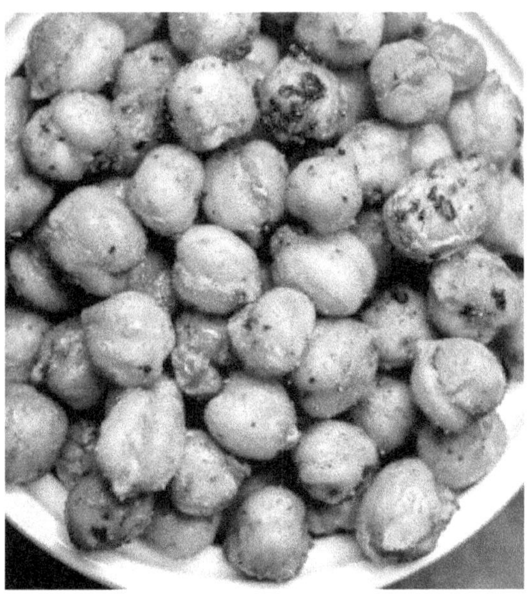

Ingredients:
- 1 can chickpeas (drained and rinsed)
- 2 tablespoons olive oil
- 1 teaspoon salt
- 1/2 teaspoon garlic powder
- 1/2 teaspoon paprika
- Optional: other spices or seasonings of your choice (e.g., cumin, chili powder, lemon zest)

Instructions:
1. Preheat the oven to 400°F (200°C).
2. Rinse the chickpeas and remove any loose skins.
3. In a bowl, mix together the olive oil, salt, garlic powder, paprika, and any desired additional spices.

4. Add the chickpeas to the bowl and toss to coat evenly with the spice mixture.
5. Spread the chickpeas on a baking sheet in a single layer.
6. Roast in the preheated oven for 30-40 minutes, or until crispy and golden brown.
7. Remove from the oven and let cool completely.

Tips:
- Use different seasonings or spices to change up the flavor.
- Try roasting chickpeas with other vegetables, like broccoli or sweet potatoes, for a tasty snack mix.
- Store roasted chickpeas in an airtight container for up to 3 days.

4. Avocado Toast

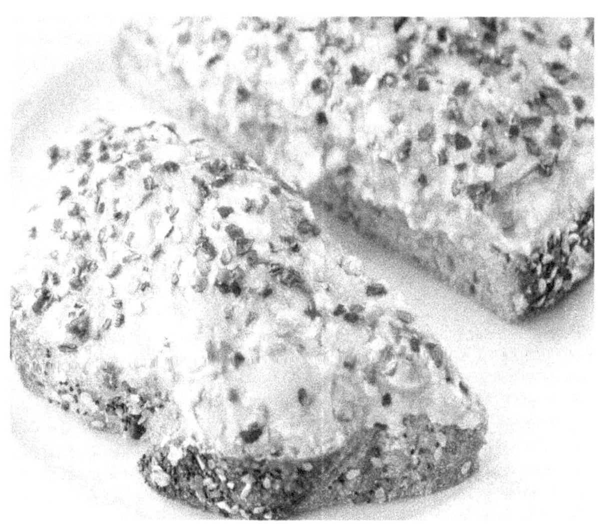

Ingredients:
- 2 slices whole grain bread
- 1 ripe avocado, mashed
- Salt and pepper to taste
- Optional: lemon juice, red pepper flakes, feta cheese, or other toppings of your choice

Instructions:
1. Toast the bread until lightly browned.
2. Spread the mashed avocado on top of the toast.
3. Sprinkle it with salt and pepper to taste.
4. Add any desired toppings, such as a squeeze of lemon juice or a sprinkle of red pepper flakes.
5. Serve and enjoy!

Tips:
- Use different types of bread, such as whole wheat or sourdough, for a varied texture and flavor.
- Add some crunch with chopped nuts or seeds, like almonds or pumpkin seeds.
- Mix in some diced tomatoes or garlic for extra flavor.
- Try using different types of cheese, like goat cheese or parmesan, for a unique twist.

5. Trail Mix

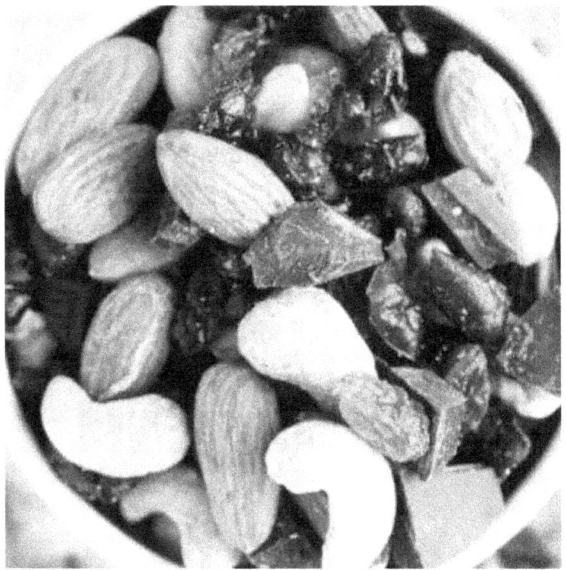

Ingredients:
- 2 cups mixed nuts (such as almonds, cashews, and walnuts)
- 1 cup dried fruit (such as cranberries, raisins, and cherries)
- 1/2 cup seeds (such as pumpkin and sunflower)
- 1/4 cup dark chocolate chips (at least 70% cocoa)
- Optional: other ingredients like coconut flakes, cinnamon, or nut butter

Instructions:
1. In a large bowl, mix together the nuts, dried fruit, and seeds.
2. Add the dark chocolate chips and any desired additional ingredients.

3. Mix until well combined.

4. Store in an airtight container for up to 2 weeks.

Tips:

- Customize the recipe with your favorite ingredients.

- Use different types of nuts or seeds for varied textures and flavors.

- Add some spice with cinnamon or nutmeg.

- Try using different types of chocolate chips or adding some cocoa nibs for extra flavor.

6. Cottage Cheese And Fresh Fruit

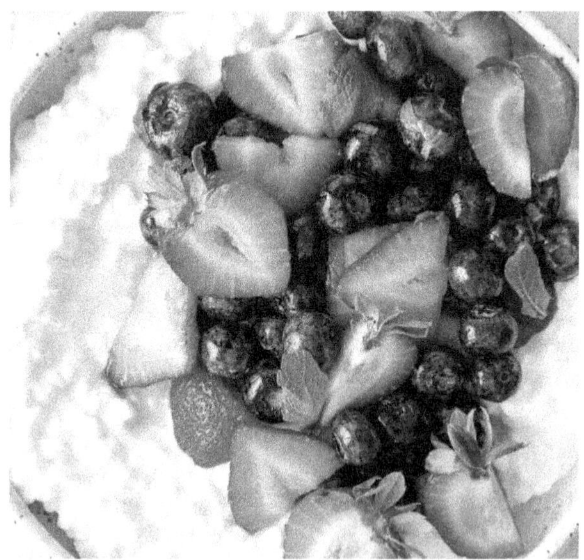

Ingredients:

- 1 cup cottage cheese

- 1/2 cup fresh fruit (such as berries, sliced peaches, or diced pineapple)
- Optional: 1 tablespoon honey or maple syrup (optional)

Instructions:

1. In a bowl, mix together the cottage cheese and fresh fruit.
2. Add a drizzle of honey or maple syrup, if desired, for a touch of sweetness.
3. Serve and enjoy!

Tips:

- Use different types of fruit to mix and match your favorite flavors and textures.
- Add some crunch with chopped nuts or seeds, like almonds or chia seeds.
- Try using different flavors of cottage cheese, like vanilla or strawberry.
- Consider adding a sprinkle of cinnamon or nutmeg for extra flavor.

7. Dark Chocolate-Dipped Fruit

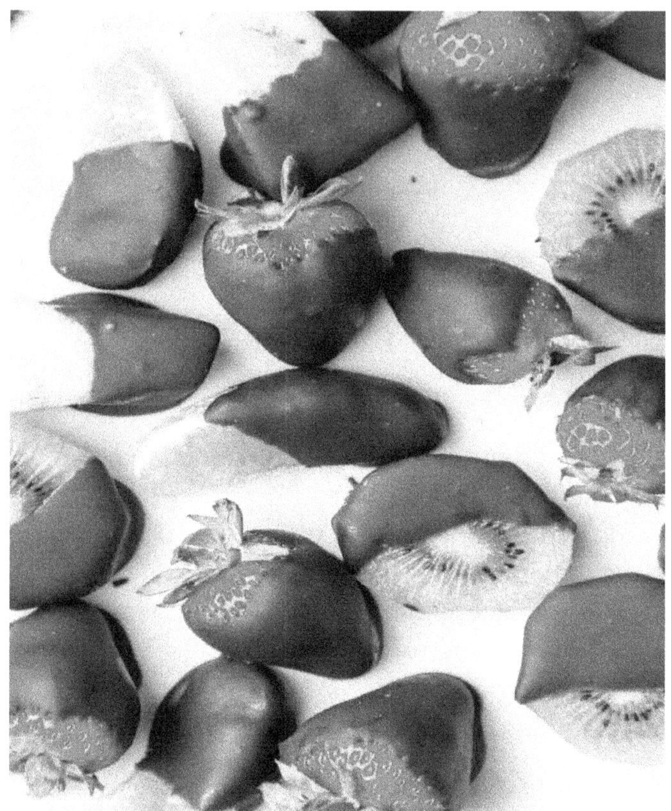

Ingredients:
- 1 cup fresh fruit (such as strawberries, bananas, or grapes)
- 1/2 cup dark chocolate chips (at least 70% cocoa)
- Optional: chopped nuts or shredded coconut for added crunch

Instructions:
1. Wash and dry the fresh fruit thoroughly.

2. Melt the dark chocolate chips in a double boiler
or in the microwave in 30-second increments,
stirring between each interval until smooth.
3. Dip each piece of fruit into the melted chocolate,
coating about half of the fruit.
4. Place the dipped fruit on a parchment-lined
baking sheet.
5. If using, sprinkle with chopped nuts or shredded
coconut before the chocolate hardens.
6. Refrigerate until the chocolate is set, about 30
minutes.
7. Enjoy your delicious and healthy snack!

Tips:
- Use different types of fruit to mix and match your
favorite flavors and textures.
- Experiment with different types of chocolate, like
white chocolate or caramel-filled chocolate chips.
- Add some spice with a sprinkle of cinnamon or
cayenne pepper.
- Consider using dried fruit, like cranberries or
apricots, for a chewy texture.

8. Energy Balls

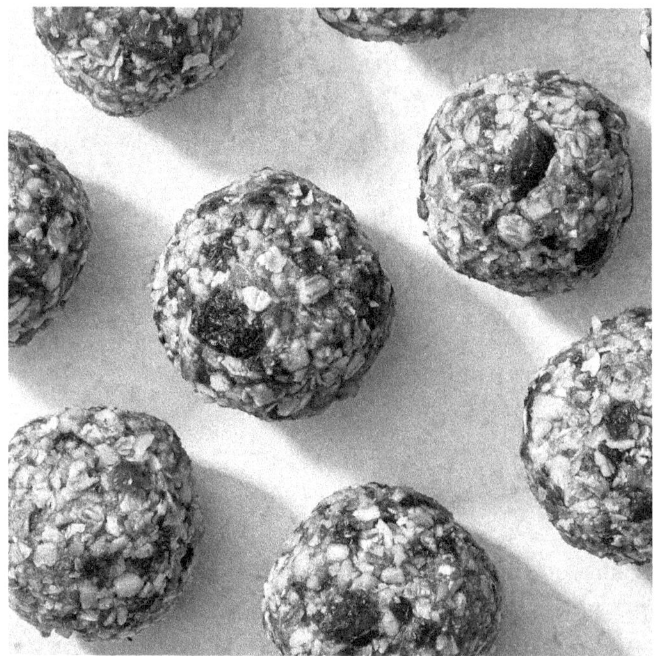

Ingredients:
- 2 cups rolled oats
- 1 cup nut butter (such as peanut butter or almond butter)
- 1/2 cup honey or maple syrup
- 1/4 cup chia seeds
- 1/4 cup shredded coconut
- Optional: chocolate chips, cinnamon, or vanilla extract

Instructions:
1. In a large bowl, combine the oats, nut butter, and honey or maple syrup. Mix until well combined.

2. Stir in the chia seeds and shredded coconut.
3. If using, add chocolate chips, cinnamon, or vanilla extract and mix until distributed.
4. Use your hands to shape the mixture into small balls, about 1 inch in diameter.
5. Place the energy balls on a parchment-lined baking sheet and refrigerate for at least 30 minutes to set.
6. Store in an airtight container in the refrigerator for up to a week.

Tips:
- Use different types of nut butter or add some nutmeg for varied flavors.
- Add some crunch with chopped nuts or seeds, like almonds or pumpkin seeds.
- Experiment with different sweeteners, like coconut sugar or dates.
- Consider using different types of oats, like steel-cut or quick-cooking oats.

9. Hummus And Veggie Sticks

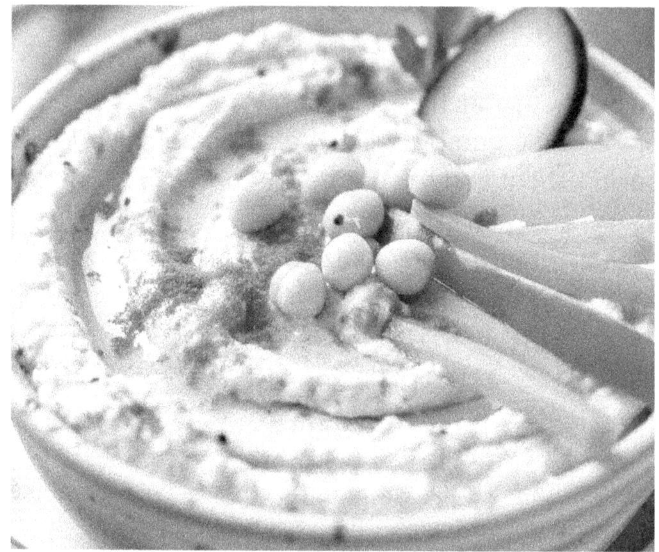

Ingredients:
- 1 cup cooked chickpeas
- 1/4 cup lemon juice
- 1/4 cup tahini
- 2 cloves garlic, minced
- 1/2 teaspoon salt
- 3 tablespoons olive oil
- Carrot sticks, celery sticks, and cucumber slices for dipping

Instructions:
1. In a blender or food processor, combine the chickpeas, lemon juice, tahini, garlic, and salt. Blend until smooth.

2. With the blender or food processor running, slowly pour in the olive oil until the hummus is creamy and smooth.
3. Taste and adjust the seasoning as needed.
4. Serve the hummus with carrot sticks, celery sticks, and cucumber slices for dipping.

Tips:
- Use different types of beans, like black beans or edamame, for a varied flavor.
- Add some spice with a pinch of cumin or paprika.
- Experiment with different herbs, like parsley or dill, for added freshness.
- Consider using different types of vinegar, like apple cider vinegar, for a unique flavor.

10. Banana Oat Bites

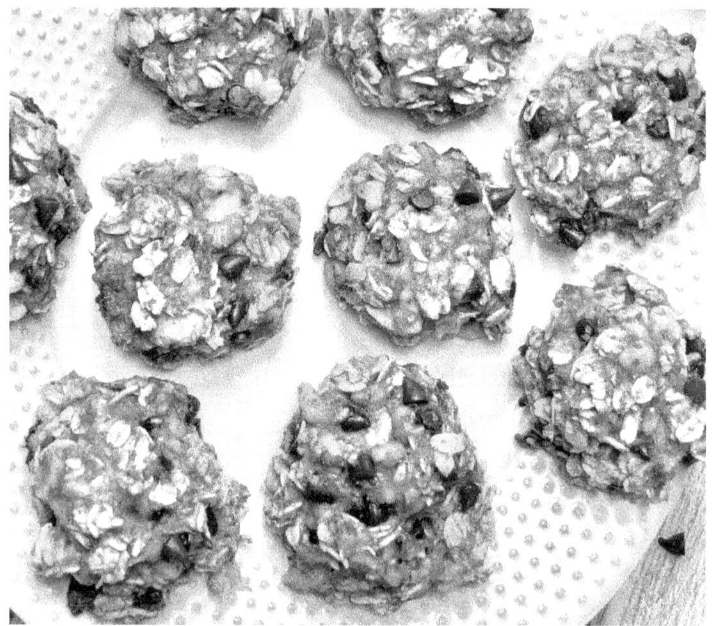

Ingredients:
- 2 ripe bananas
- 1/2 cup rolled oats
- 1/4 cup nut butter (like peanut butter or almond butter)
- 1/4 cup honey or maple syrup
- 1/4 cup chopped nuts (like walnuts or almonds)
- Pinch of salt

Instructions:
1. In a bowl, mash the bananas with a fork until smooth.
2. Add the oats, nut butter, honey or maple syrup, chopped nuts, and salt. Mix until well combined.

3. Use your hands to shape the mixture into small balls, about 1 inch in diameter.
4. Place the banana oat bites on a parchment-lined baking sheet and refrigerate for at least 30 minutes to set.
5. Store in an airtight container in the refrigerator for up to 5 days.

Tips:
- Use different types of nut butter or add some cinnamon for varied flavors.
- Add some chocolate chips for a sweet surprise.
- Experiment with different types of oats, like steel-cut or quick-cooking oats.
- Consider using different types of nuts, like pecans or hazelnuts, for added crunch.

Energizing Drinks

1. Berry Bliss Smoothie

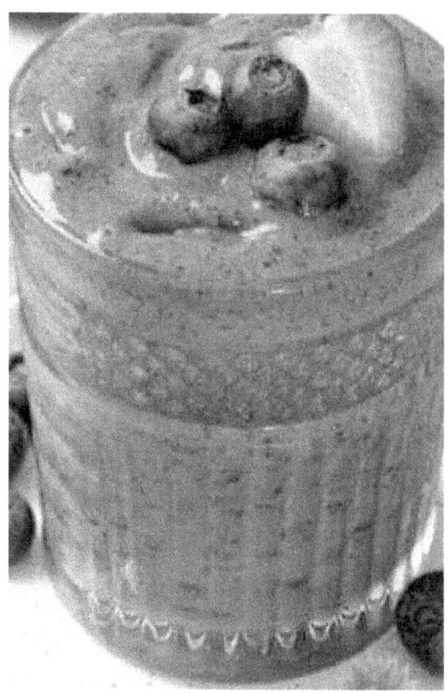

Ingredients:
- 1 cup frozen mixed berries (blueberries, strawberries, raspberries)
- 1/2 cup fresh spinach leaves
- 1/2 cup unsweetened almond milk
- 1 tablespoon chia seeds
- 1 teaspoon honey (optional)

Instructions:

1. Add all the ingredients to a blender and blend until smooth.
2. Taste and adjust the sweetness by adding more honey if needed.
3. Pour into a glass and serve immediately.

2. Cinnamon Apple Cider

Ingredients:
- 2 cups apple cider
- 1 cinnamon stick
- 1/4 teaspoon ground cinnamon
- 1/4 teaspoon ground nutmeg
- 1/4 teaspoon ground ginger
- 1 tablespoon honey (optional)
- Lemon slices or cinnamon sticks for garnish (optional)

Instructions:
1. In a medium saucepan, heat the apple cider over medium heat until warm.
2. Add the cinnamon stick, ground cinnamon, nutmeg, and ginger.
3. Reduce heat and simmer for 5-7 minutes.
4. Strain into mugs and discard solids.
5. Add honey to taste, if desired.
6. Garnish with lemon slices or cinnamon sticks, if desired.

3. Green Goddess Juice

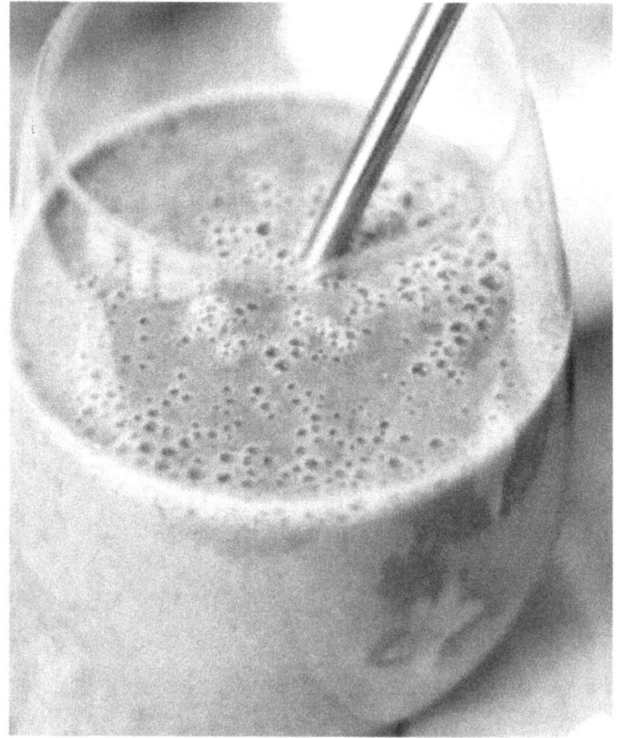

Ingredients:

- 2 cups kale, stems removed and discarded, leaves coarsely chopped
- 1 cup fresh green apple, cored and chopped
- 1/2 cup fresh celery, chopped
- 1/2 cup fresh cucumber, peeled and chopped
- 1/4 cup fresh lemon juice
- 1/4 cup fresh ginger, peeled and chopped
- Ice cubes (optional)

Instructions:

1. Add all the ingredients to a juicer or blender and juice or blend until smooth.
2. Strain the juice through a fine-mesh sieve into a large bowl or pitcher.
3. Discard the solids and serve the juice immediately.
4. Add ice cubes if you prefer a chilled juice.

4. Turmeric Ginger Latte

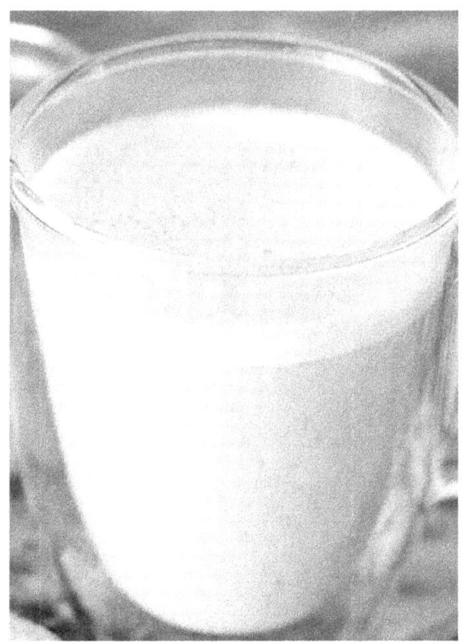

Ingredients:
- 1 cup non-dairy milk (almond, coconut, or oat milk)
- 1 teaspoon turmeric powder
- 1/2 teaspoon ground ginger

- 1/2 teaspoon honey or maple syrup (optional)
- 1/4 teaspoon ground cinnamon (optional)
- 1/4 teaspoon ground black pepper (optional)

Instructions:

1. In a small saucepan, warm the non-dairy milk over medium heat.
2. Add the turmeric, ginger, honey or maple syrup (if using), cinnamon (if using), and black pepper (if using).
3. Whisk until the mixture is smooth and warm.
4. Pour into a mug and serve immediately.

5. Raspberry Leaf Tea

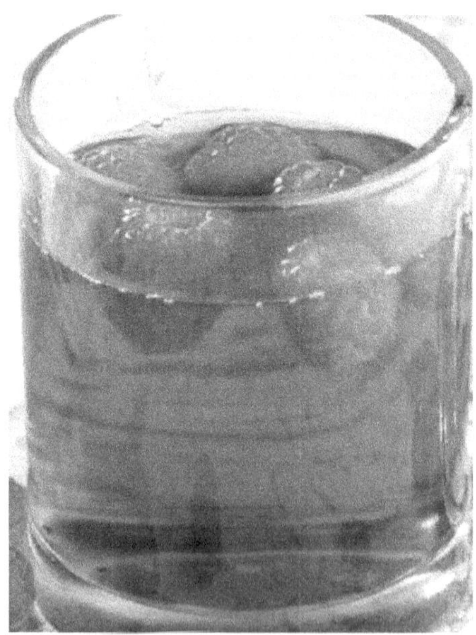

Ingredients:

- 1 cup dried raspberry leaves
- 1 cup boiling water
- 1 tablespoon honey (optional)
- Lemon slices or fresh raspberries for garnish
(optional)

Instructions:
1. Pour boiling water over the dried raspberry
leaves in a teapot or infuser.
2. Let it steep for 5-7 minutes, then strain into a
cup.
3. Add honey to taste, if desired.
4. Garnish with lemon slices or fresh raspberries, if
desired.

Raspberry leaf tea is a herbal tea that's rich in
nutrients and has several health benefits, including:

- Supporting menstrual health and fertility
- Easing pregnancy symptoms like morning
sickness and cramps
- Providing antioxidants and anti-inflammatory
properties

Note: Consult with a healthcare professional before
consuming raspberry leaf tea, especially if you're
pregnant or have any underlying health conditions.

6. Peachy Keen Smoothie

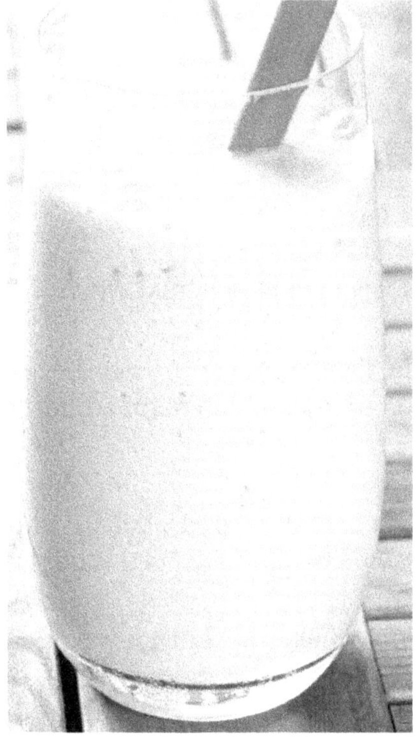

Ingredients:
- 1 ripe peach, diced
- 1/2 cup plain Greek yogurt
- 1/2 cup unsweetened almond milk
- 1 tablespoon honey
- 1/2 teaspoon vanilla extract
- Ice cubes (optional)

Instructions:
1. Add all the ingredients to a blender and blend until smooth.

2. Taste and adjust the sweetness or consistency as needed.
3. Add ice cubes if you want a thicker, colder smoothie.
4. Blend again until the ice is crushed and the smoothie is the desired consistency.
5. Pour into a glass and serve immediately.

7. Cranberry Lime Spritzer

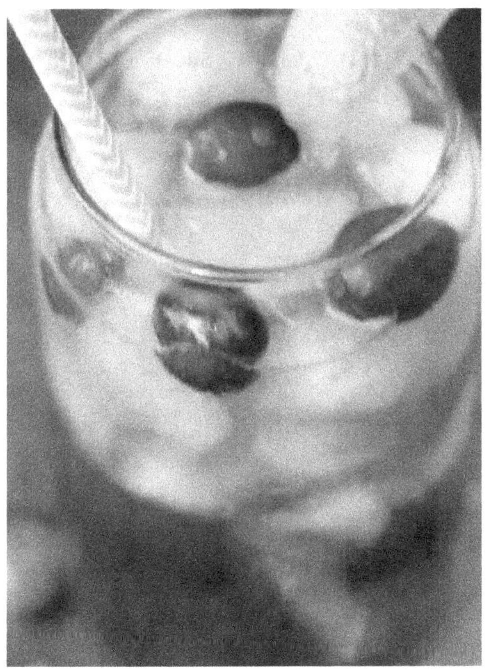

Ingredients:
- 2 cups cranberry juice (unsweetened or low-sugar)
- 1/2 cup fresh lime juice

- 1/4 cup sparkling water
- 1/4 cup ice
- Lime slices or fresh cranberries for garnish
(optional)

Instructions:
1. In a large pitcher, mix together cranberry juice
and lime juice.
2. Add sparkling water and stir well.
3. Fill glasses with ice and pour the Cranberry Lime
Spritzer over the ice.
4. Stir gently and garnish with lime slices or fresh
cranberries, if desired.

8. Ginger Pear Juice

Ingredients:
- 2 ripe pears, cored and chopped
- 1-inch piece of fresh ginger, peeled and chopped
- 1 cup water
- 1/4 cup honey (optional)
- Ice cubes (optional)

Instructions:
1. In a blender or juicer, combine pears, ginger, and
water.
2. Blend or juice until smooth.
3. Strain the mixture through a fine-mesh sieve into
a large bowl or pitcher.
4. Discard the solids.
5. Add honey to taste, if desired, and stir well.

6. Serve immediately, or chill in the refrigerator for later.
7. Add ice cubes, if desired, and serve.

9. Chamomile Citrus Tea

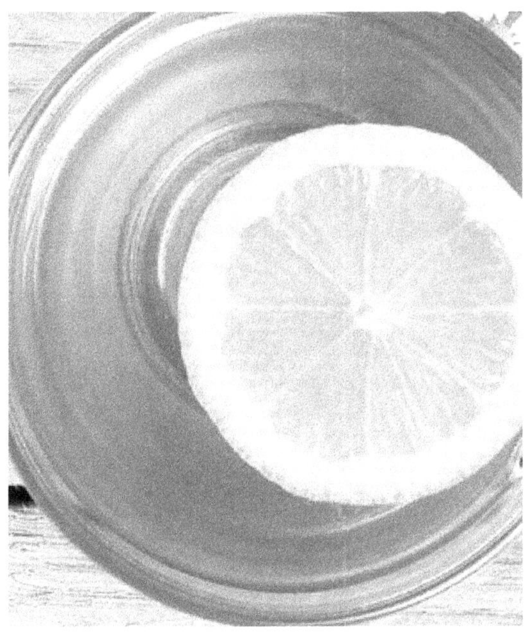

Ingredients:
- 1 teaspoon dried chamomile flowers
- 1 teaspoon dried citrus peel (orange or lemon)
- 1 cup boiling water
- 1 tablespoon honey (optional)
- Lemon slices or citrus wedges for garnish (optional)

Instructions:

1. In a tea infuser or a heat-resistant cup, combine chamomile flowers and citrus peel.
2. Pour boiling water over the mixture and let it steep for 5-7 minutes.
3. Strain the tea into a cup and discard the solids.
4. Add honey to taste, if desired.
5. Garnish with lemon slices or citrus wedges, if desired.

10. Beetroot Blast Smoothie

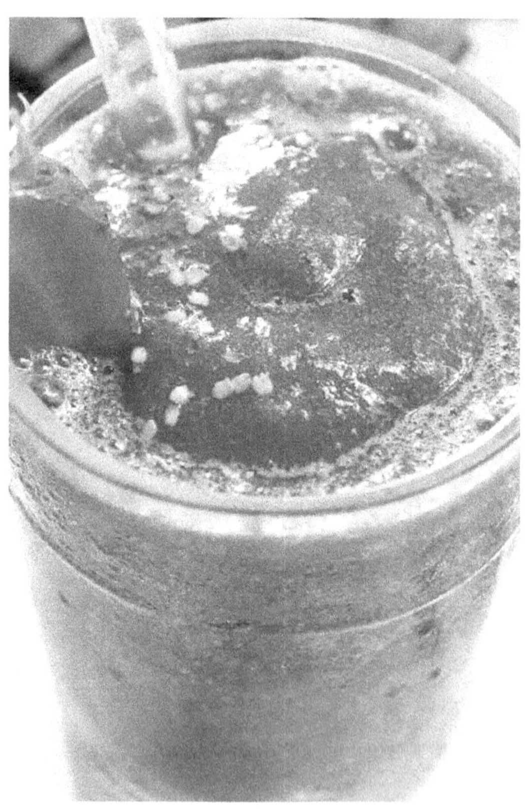

Ingredients:
- 2 medium beetroot, peeled and chopped
- 1/2 cup frozen pineapple
- 1/2 cup frozen berries (blueberries, strawberries, or raspberries)
- 1/2 cup plain Greek yogurt
- 1/2 cup unsweetened almond milk
- 1 tablespoon honey (optional)
- Ice cubes (optional)

Instructions:
1. Add all the ingredients to a blender and blend until smooth.
2. Taste and adjust the sweetness or consistency as needed.
3. Add ice cubes if you want a thicker, colder smoothie.
4. Blend again until the ice is crushed and the smoothie is the desired consistency.
5. Pour into a glass and serve immediately.

This smoothie is a vibrant and healthy blend of beetroot, pineapple, and berries. The beetroot provides a boost of antioxidants and fiber, while the Greek yogurt adds protein and creaminess.

Chapter Five

Special Diets And Considerations

- Focus on whole, unprocessed foods
- Include lean protein sources like poultry, fish, and legumes
- Choose complex carbohydrates like whole grains, fruits, and vegetables
- Healthy fats like avocado, nuts, and olive oil are encouraged
- Limit processed and high-sugar foods
- Stay hydrated by drinking plenty of water
- Consider working with a registered dietitian for personalized guidance

Gluten Free And Grain Free Recipes

1. Quinoa Salad

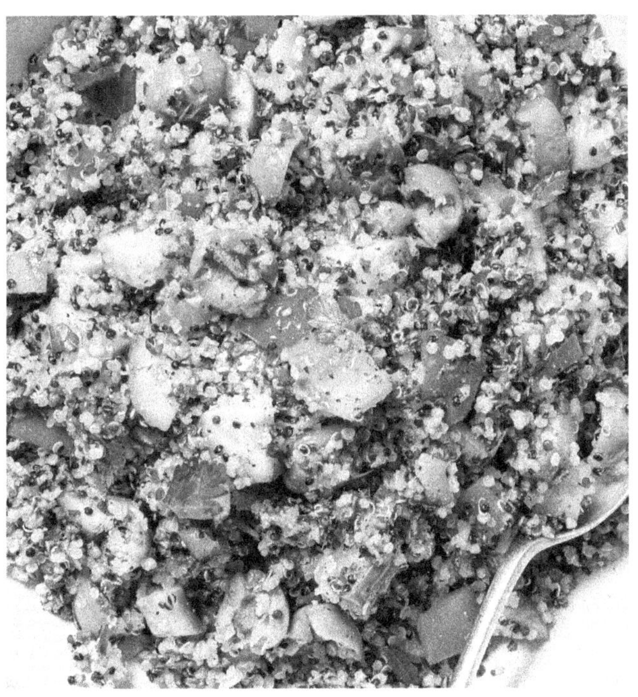

Ingredients:
- 1 cup quinoa, rinsed and drained
- 2 cups water or vegetable broth
- 2 cups mixed vegetables (bell peppers, cucumbers, cherry tomatoes, carrots)
- 1/4 cup fresh parsley, chopped
- 2 tablespoons lemon juice

- 1 tablespoon olive oil
- Salt and pepper to taste
- 1/4 teaspoon paprika (optional)

Instructions:
1. Rinse quinoa and cook according to package instructions.
2. In a large bowl, combine cooked quinoa, mixed vegetables, parsley, lemon juice, olive oil, salt, pepper, and paprika (if using).
3. Toss to combine and adjust seasoning as needed.
4. Serve chilled or at room temperature.

Note: You can customize the recipe by adding your favorite vegetables, nuts, or protein sources like grilled chicken or tofu.

2. Grilled Chicken And Vegetable Skewers

Ingredients:
- 1 pound boneless, skinless chicken breast or thighs, cut into 1-inch pieces
- 1 cup mixed vegetables (bell peppers, onions, mushrooms, cherry tomatoes, zucchini)
- 2 tablespoons olive oil
- 1 tablespoon lemon juice
- 1 clove garlic, minced
- 1 teaspoon dried oregano
- Salt and pepper to taste

Instructions:

1. Preheat the grill to medium-high heat.
2. Thread chicken and vegetables onto skewers.
3. In a small bowl, whisk together olive oil, lemon juice, garlic, and oregano.
4. Brush the mixture onto both sides of the skewers.
5. Season with salt and pepper to taste.
6. Grill for 10-12 minutes or until chicken is cooked through and vegetables are tender.
7. Serve hot with your favorite side dish or salad.

3. Buckwheat Pancakes

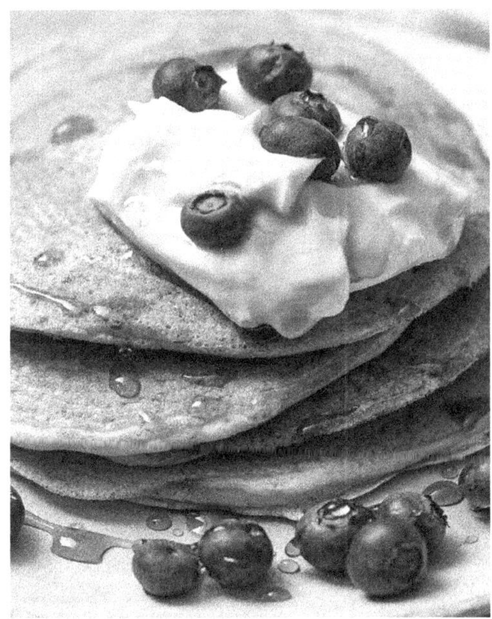

Ingredients:

- 1 cup buckwheat flour
- 2 cups almond milk
- 1/4 cup honey or maple syrup
- 1 large egg
- 1/4 teaspoon salt
- 1/4 teaspoon baking powder
- 2 tablespoons melted coconut oil
- Fresh fruit or nuts for topping (optional)

Instructions:

1. In a large bowl, whisk together buckwheat flour, almond milk, honey or maple syrup, egg, salt, and baking powder.
2. Add melted coconut oil and whisk until smooth.
3. Heat a non-stick skillet or griddle over medium heat.
4. Drop batter by 1/4 cupfuls onto the skillet or griddle.
5. Cook for 2-3 minutes or until bubbles appear on the surface and edges start to dry.
6. Flip and cook for another 1-2 minutes or until golden brown.
7. Serve warm with fresh fruit or nuts, if desired.

Note: Buckwheat flour has a distinct nutty flavor and a denser texture than regular pancakes. You can adjust the recipe by adding different spices or sweeteners to taste.

4. Cauliflower Fried Rice

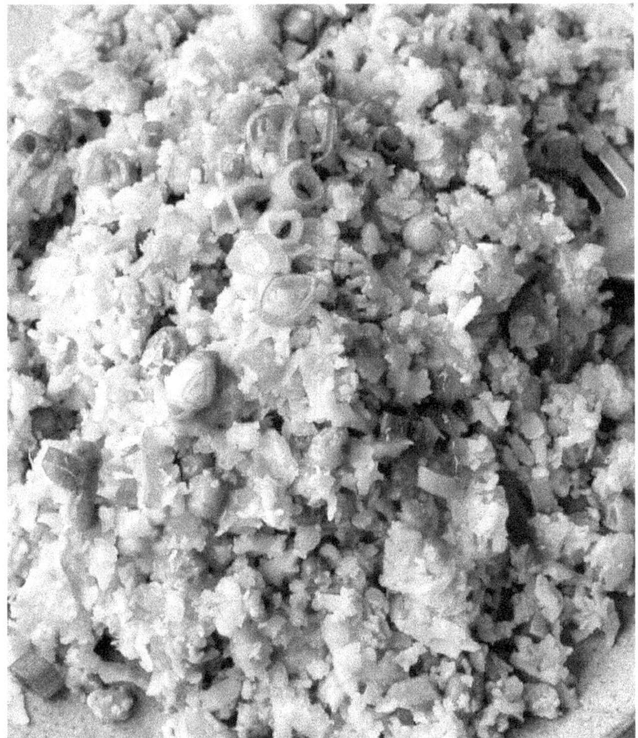

Ingredients:
- 1 head of cauliflower
- 2 cups cooked rice (preferably day-old rice)
- 1 tablespoon coconut oil
- 1 small onion, diced
- 2 cloves garlic, minced
- 1 cup mixed vegetables (e.g., peas, carrots, corn)
- 2 eggs, beaten
- 1 teaspoon soy sauce
- Salt and pepper to taste
- Scallions for garnish (optional)

Instructions:
1. Pulse cauliflower in a food processor until it resembles rice.
2. Heat coconut oil in a large skillet or wok over medium-high heat.
3. Add onion and garlic and cook until softened.
4. Add mixed vegetables and cook until tender.
5. Push vegetables to one side of the pan.
6. Add beaten eggs and scramble until cooked through.
7. Mix eggs with vegetables.
8. Add cauliflower "rice" and cooked rice to the pan.
9. Stir-fry everything together.
10. Add soy sauce and season with salt and pepper to taste.
11. Garnish with scallions (if using) and serve hot.

5. Grilled Salmon With Roasted Vegetables

Ingredients:
- 4 salmon filets (6 ounces each)
- 2 cups mixed vegetables (asparagus, Brussels sprouts, red bell peppers, zucchini)
- 2 tablespoons olive oil
- 1 tablespoon lemon juice
- 1 clove garlic, minced
- Salt and pepper to taste

Instructions:

1. Preheat the grill to medium-high heat.
2. Season salmon filets with salt, pepper, and garlic.
3. Grill salmon for 4-6 minutes per side or until cooked through.
4. Toss vegetables with olive oil, salt, and pepper.
5. Spread vegetables on a baking sheet and roast in the oven at 425°F (220°C) for 15-20 minutes or until tender.
6. Serve grilled salmon with roasted vegetables and a squeeze of lemon juice.

6. Zucchini Noodles With Meat Sauce

Ingredients:
- 2 medium zucchinis
- 1 pound ground meat (beef, pork, or turkey)
- 1 onion, diced

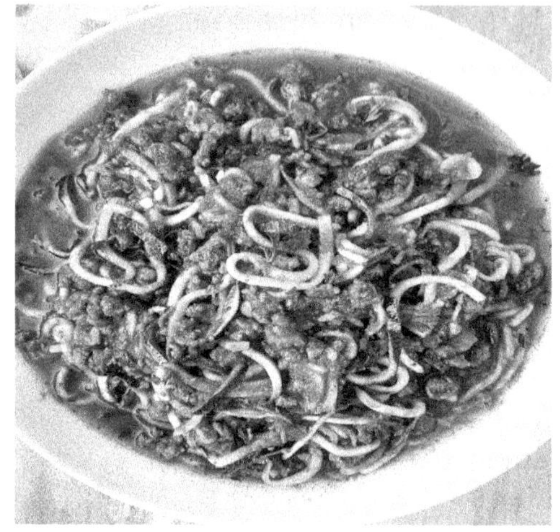

- 2 cloves garlic, minced
- 1 cup tomato sauce
- 1 cup beef broth
- 1 tablespoon olive oil
- Salt and pepper to taste
- Optional: 1/4 cup grated Parmesan cheese

Instructions:
1. Spiralize zucchini into noodles.
2. Cook ground meat in a large skillet over medium-high heat until browned, breaking it up into small pieces.
3. Add onion and garlic to the skillet and cook until softened.
4. Add tomato sauce, beef broth, and olive oil to the skillet. Stir to combine.
5. Bring the sauce to a simmer and let cook for 5-7 minutes or until slightly thickened.
6. Add zucchini noodles to the skillet and toss with the meat sauce.

7. Season with salt and pepper to taste.
8. Serve hot, topped with Parmesan cheese if desired.

7. Stuffed Bell Peppers

Ingredients:
- 4 bell peppers, any color
- 1 pound ground meat (beef, pork, or turkey)
- 1 onion, diced
- 2 cloves garlic, minced
- 1 cup cooked rice
- 1 cup black beans, drained and rinsed
- 1 cup diced tomatoes
- 1 teaspoon cumin
- 1/2 teaspoon paprika
- Salt and pepper to taste
- 1/4 cup shredded cheese (optional)

Instructions:
1. Preheat the oven to 375°F (190°C).
2. Cut the tops off the bell peppers and remove seeds and membranes.
3. Cook ground meat in a large skillet over medium-high heat until browned, breaking it up into small pieces.
4. Add onion, garlic, cooked rice, black beans, diced tomatoes, cumin, paprika, salt, and pepper to the skillet. Stir to combine.
5. Stuff each bell pepper with the meat mixture and top with shredded cheese (if using).

6. Place bell peppers in a baking dish and cover with a lid or foil.
7. Bake for 25-30 minutes or until bell peppers are tender.
8. Serve hot and enjoy!

8. Chicken Soup And Cabbage

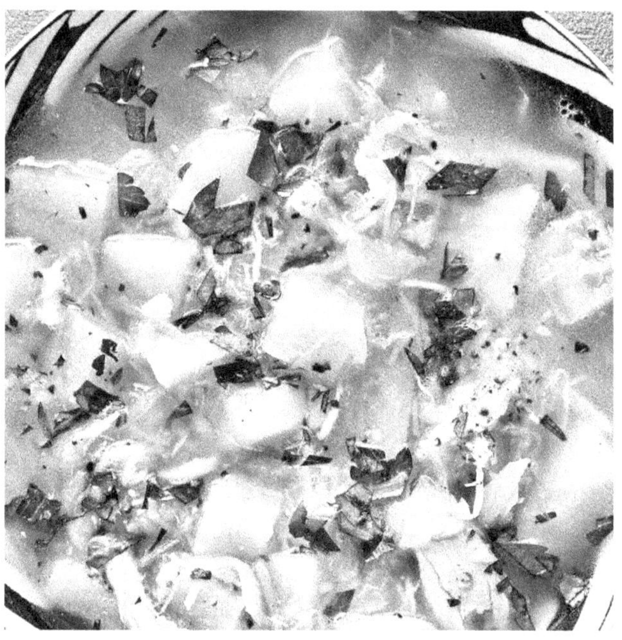

Ingredients:
- 1 pound boneless, skinless chicken breast or thighs
- 2 cups chicken broth (make sure it's low-sodium and sugar-free)
- 1 medium onion, chopped
- 3 cloves garlic, minced

- 1 medium cabbage, chopped
- 2 carrots, peeled and chopped
- 2 celery stalks, chopped
- 1 teaspoon dried thyme
- Salt and pepper, to taste
- 2 tablespoons olive oil (optional)

Instructions:
1. In a large pot, sauté the chopped onion, garlic, carrots, and celery in olive oil until tender.
2. Add the chicken and cook until browned.
3. Pour in the chicken broth, thyme, salt, and pepper. Bring to a boil, then reduce heat and let simmer.
4. Add the chopped cabbage and continue to simmer until the vegetables are tender and the chicken is cooked through.
5. Serve hot and enjoy!

9. Vegetable Stir-Fry With Tofu

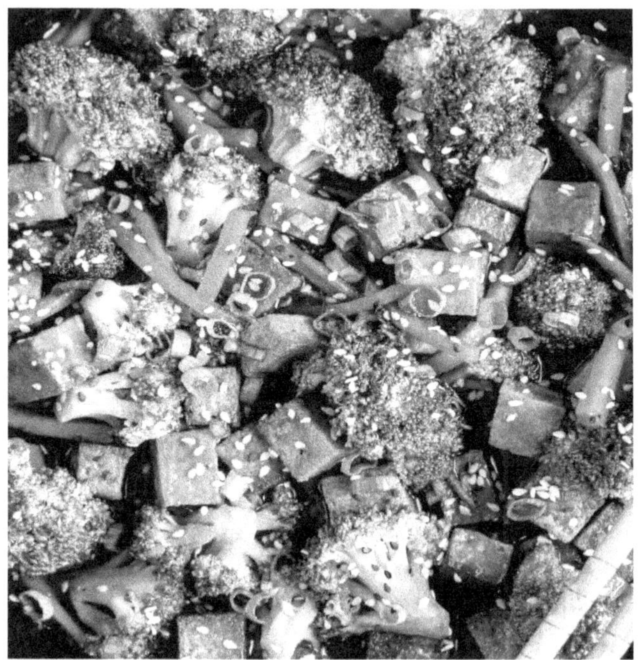

Ingredients:
- 1 cup firm tofu, cut into small cubes
- 2 cups mixed vegetables (broccoli, bell peppers, carrots, snap peas, mushrooms)
- 2 tablespoons olive oil
- 1 tablespoon soy sauce
- 1 tablespoon honey
- 1 clove garlic, minced
- 1 teaspoon grated ginger
- Salt and pepper to taste
- Optional: sesame seeds and green onions for garnish

Instructions:

1. Heat olive oil in a large skillet or wok over medium-high heat.
2. Add tofu and cook until golden brown, about 3-4 minutes per side.
3. Add mixed vegetables, soy sauce, honey, garlic, and ginger to the skillet.
4. Stir-fry for 4-5 minutes or until vegetables are tender-crisp.
5. Return tofu to the skillet and stir to combine.
6. Season with salt and pepper to taste.
7. Garnish with sesame seeds and green onions (if using).
8. Serve hot over rice or noodles.

10. Coconut Flour Bread

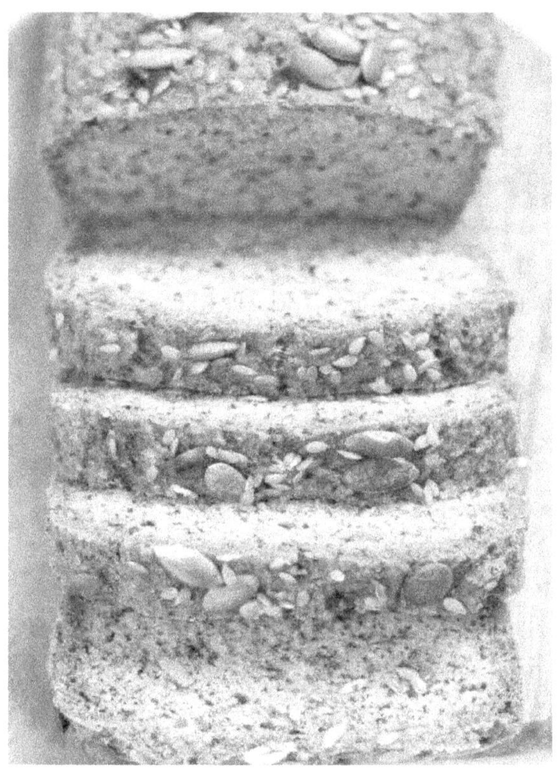

Ingredients:

- 1 1/2 cups coconut flour
- 1/4 cup coconut oil, melted
- 1/4 cup honey or maple syrup
- 3 large eggs
- 1/2 teaspoon salt
- 1 teaspoon baking soda
- 1 teaspoon vanilla extract
- Optional: nuts, seeds, or dried fruit for added texture and flavor

Instructions:
1. Preheat the oven to 350°F (180°C). Grease a 9x5-inch loaf pan.
2. In a large bowl, combine coconut flour, melted coconut oil, honey or maple syrup, eggs, salt, baking soda, and vanilla extract.
3. Mix well until a sticky dough forms.
4. Add optional nuts, seeds, or dried fruit (if using).
5. Pour dough into the prepared loaf pan and smooth the top.
6. Bake for 35-40 minutes or until a toothpick inserted into the center comes out clean.
7. Let cool on a wire rack for 10 minutes before slicing and serving.

Note: Coconut flour absorbs liquid differently than traditional flour, so the texture may be denser. You can adjust the recipe by adding more eggs or honey to achieve your desired consistency.

Vegetarian And Vegan Recipes

1. Vegan Jackfruit Tacos With Turmeric Slaw

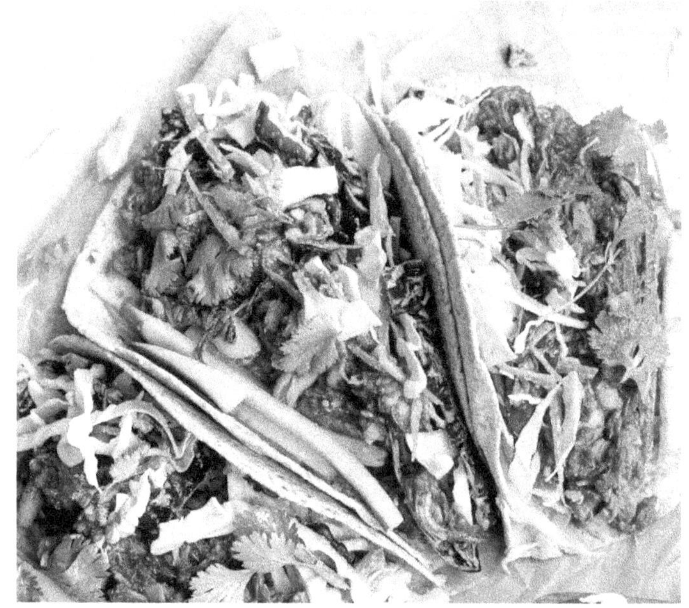

Ingredients:
- 1 cup jackfruit (canned or fresh)
- 1/2 cup turmeric slaw (made with red cabbage, carrots, and turmeric)
- 1/4 cup lime juice
- 1/4 cup chopped cilantro
- 1 jalapeno pepper, sliced
- 6 corn tortillas

- Salt and pepper, to taste

Instructions:
1. Drain and rinse the jackfruit, then shred it with a fork.
2. In a pan, heat some oil and sauté the jackfruit with lime juice, cilantro, and jalapeno until tender.
3. Warm the tortillas by wrapping them in a damp paper towel and microwaving for 20-30 seconds.
4. Assemble the tacos by filling the tortillas with the jackfruit mixture and topping with turmeric slaw.
5. Serve immediately and enjoy!

The turmeric slaw adds a nice crunch and a boost of anti-inflammatory properties from the turmeric.

2. Stuffed Delicata Squash With Wild Rice And Mushrooms

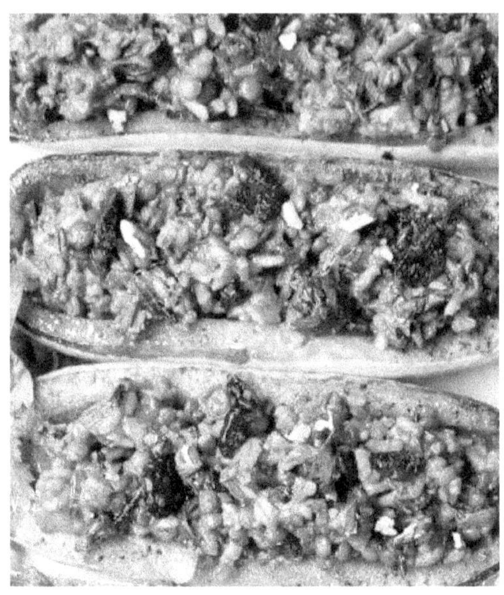

Ingredients:
- 2 delicata squash, halved and seeds removed
- 1 cup wild rice, cooked
- 1 cup mixed mushrooms (such as cremini, shiitake, and oyster), sliced
- 2 tablespoons olive oil
- 1 onion, chopped
- 2 cloves garlic, minced
- 1 teaspoon dried thyme
- Salt and pepper, to taste

Instructions:
1. Preheat the oven to 400°F (200°C).

2. In a pan, heat oil and sauté the onion, garlic, and mushrooms until tender.
3. Add the cooked wild rice, thyme, salt, and pepper to the pan and stir to combine.
4. Divide the rice mixture among the squash halves, filling them generously.
5. Bake for 30-40 minutes or until the squash is tender and the filling is heated through.
6. Serve warm and enjoy.

3. Lentil And Vegetable Koftas With Tzatziki Sauce

Ingredients:
- 1 cup cooked lentils
- 1 cup mixed vegetables (such as carrots, zucchini, and bell peppers)
- 1/2 cup breadcrumbs
- 1 egg, lightly beaten
- 1 tablespoon olive oil
- 1 onion, finely chopped
- 2 cloves garlic, minced
- 1 teaspoon cumin
- Salt and pepper, to taste
- Tzatziki sauce (made with yogurt, cucumber, garlic, and dill)

Instructions:
1. Preheat the oven to 375°F (190°C).

2. In a food processor, blend the lentils, vegetables, breadcrumbs, egg, oil, onion, garlic, cumin, salt, and pepper until well combined.
3. Shape the mixture into small cylinders and place on a baking sheet lined with parchment paper.
4. Bake for 20-25 minutes or until the koftas are firm and lightly browned.
5. Serve with tzatziki sauce for a refreshing and tangy contrast.

These koftas are a great source of plant-based protein, fiber, and vitamins, making them a nutritious addition to a PCOS diet. The tzatziki sauce adds a cool and creamy element, perfect for hot summer days.

4. Vegan Spiralized Sweet Potato And Black Bean Tacos

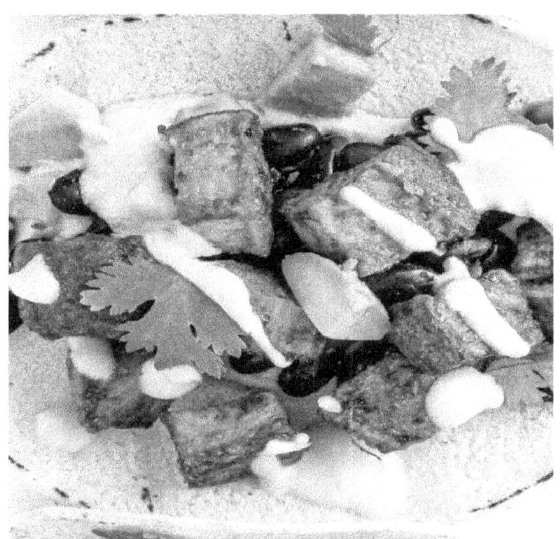

Ingredients:
- 2 large sweet potatoes, peeled and spiralized
- 1 can black beans, drained and rinsed
- 1/4 cup lime juice
- 1/4 cup chopped cilantro
- 1 jalapeno pepper, sliced
- 1 avocado, sliced (optional)
- 6 corn tortillas
- Salt and pepper, to taste

Instructions:
1. In a pan, heat some oil and sauté the spiralized sweet potatoes until tender.
2. Add the black beans, lime juice, cilantro, and jalapeno to the pan and stir to combine.

3. Warm the tortillas by wrapping them in a damp paper towel and microwaving for 20-30 seconds.
4. Assemble the tacos by filling the tortillas with the sweet potato and black bean mixture.
5. Top with sliced avocado, if desired, and serve immediately.

5. Grilled Portobello Mushroom Burgers With Caramelized Onions

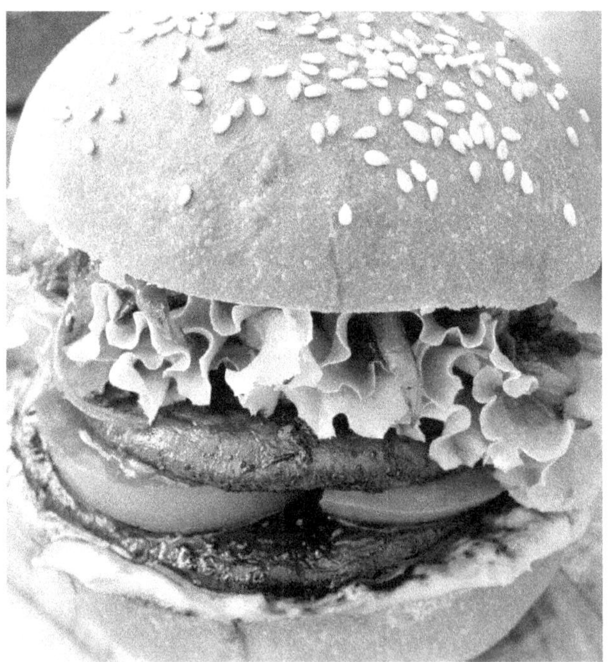

Ingredients:

- 4 Portobello mushrooms, stems removed and caps sliced 1-inch thick
- 2 tablespoons olive oil
- 1 large onion, sliced
- 2 cloves garlic, minced
- 1 tablespoon balsamic vinegar
- 1 teaspoon dried thyme
- Salt and pepper, to taste
- 4 whole-grain hamburger buns
- Lettuce, tomato, and your favorite burger toppings

Instructions:
1. In a pan, heat oil and sauté the onions and garlic until caramelized.
2. In a separate pan, grill the mushroom slices until tender and slightly charred.
3. Add the balsamic vinegar and thyme to the mushrooms and stir to combine.
4. Assemble the burgers by placing the mushrooms on the buns and topping with caramelized onions, lettuce, tomato, and your favorite toppings.

These mushroom burgers are a great source of plant-based protein, fiber, and antioxidants, making them a nutritious and delicious option for a PCOS diet. The caramelized onions add a sweet and savory flavor, while the whole-grain buns provide a good source of complex carbohydrates.

6. Vegan Butternut Squash And Sage Risotto

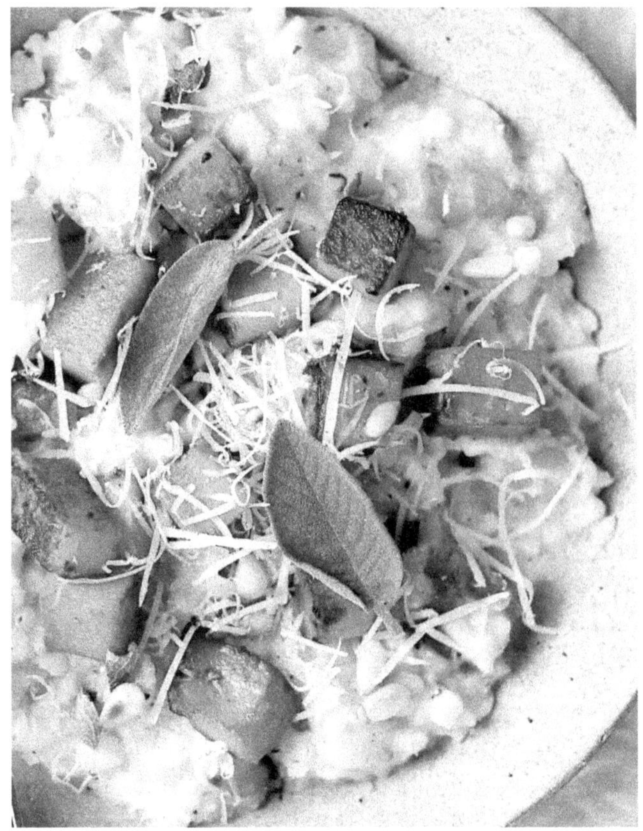

Ingredients:
- 1 medium butternut squash, peeled and cubed
- 2 tablespoons olive oil
- 1 onion, chopped
- 2 cloves garlic, minced
- 1 cup Arborio rice
- 4 cups vegetable broth, warmed

- 1 tablespoon dried sage
- Salt and pepper, to taste
- 1/4 cup vegan Parmesan cheese (optional)

Instructions:
1. Roast the butternut squash in the oven until tender.
2. In a pan, sauté the onion and garlic until softened.
3. Add the Arborio rice and cook until lightly toasted.
4. Add the warmed broth, one cup at a time, stirring continuously until the rice is cooked and creamy.
5. Stir in the roasted butternut squash, sage, salt, and pepper.
6. Serve hot, topped with vegan Parmesan cheese if desired.

This vegan butternut squash and sage risotto is a delicious and comforting meal that's perfect for a chilly evening. The roasted butternut squash adds natural sweetness, while the sage provides a savory and aromatic flavor.

7. Quinoa And Black Bean Empanadas With Chimichurri Sauce

Ingredients:
- 1 cup quinoa, cooked
- 1 cup black beans, cooked

- 1 onion, chopped
- 2 cloves garlic, minced
- 1 egg, lightly beaten
- 1 tablespoon olive oil
- 2 cups all-purpose flour
- 1 teaspoon salt
- 1/4 teaspoon black pepper
- 1/4 cup chimichurri sauce (made with parsley, oregano, garlic, red pepper flakes, red wine vinegar, and olive oil)

Instructions:
1. In a pan, sauté the onion and garlic until softened.
2. Add the cooked quinoa and black beans, and stir to combine.
3. Add the egg and stir until the mixture is well combined.
4. In a separate bowl, combine the flour, salt, and pepper.
5. Add the olive oil and chimichurri sauce to the flour mixture, and stir until a dough forms.
6. Roll out the dough and cut into circles.
7. Place a spoonful of the quinoa and black bean mixture onto each circle, and fold the dough in half to form a half-moon shape.
8. Brush the tops with egg wash and bake until golden brown.

8. Stuffed Bell Peppers With Quinoa, Mushrooms And Lentils

Ingredients:
- 4 bell peppers, any color
- 1 cup quinoa, cooked
- 1 cup lentils, cooked
- 1 cup mixed mushrooms, sliced
- 1 onion, chopped
- 2 cloves garlic, minced
- 1 tomato, diced
- 2 tablespoons olive oil
- 1 teaspoon cumin
- 1 teaspoon paprika
- Salt and pepper, to taste

Instructions:
1. Preheat the oven to 375°F (190°C).
2. Cut the tops off the bell peppers and remove seeds and membranes.
3. In a pan, sauté the onion, garlic, and mushrooms until softened.
4. Add the cooked quinoa, lentils, tomato, cumin, paprika, salt, and pepper. Stir to combine.
5. Stuff each bell pepper with the quinoa mixture and top with the pepper top.
6. Bake for 25-30 minutes or until the bell peppers are tender.

These stuffed bell peppers are a great source of plant-based protein, fiber, and vitamins, making them a nutritious and delicious option for a PCOS diet. The quinoa and lentils provide a boost of protein and fiber, while the mushrooms add a savory and earthy flavor.

9. Vegan Eggplant Parmesan With Cashew Mozzarella

Ingredients:
- 2 eggplants, sliced
- 1 cup cashews
- 1/2 cup water
- 1 tablespoon lemon juice
- 1 teaspoon apple cider vinegar
- 1/2 teaspoon salt
- 1/4 teaspoon black pepper
- 1 cup tomato sauce
- 1 cup breadcrumbs (gluten-free)
- 1/4 cup olive oil

Instructions:
1. Preheat the oven to 400°F (200°C).
2. In a blender, combine cashews, water, lemon juice, apple cider vinegar, salt, and pepper. Blend until smooth.
3. In a separate bowl, mix together tomato sauce and breadcrumbs.
4. Dip each eggplant slice into the tomato sauce mixture, then coat with the cashew mozzarella.
5. Place the eggplant slices on a baking sheet lined with parchment paper. Drizzle with olive oil.

6. Bake for 25-30 minutes or until the eggplant is tender and the cashew mozzarella is melted and golden brown.

This vegan eggplant parmesan is a game-changer for plant-based Italian cuisine. The cashew mozzarella adds a creamy and rich texture, while the eggplant provides a meaty and satisfying bite.

10. Vegan Chocolate Chia Pudding With Coconut Whipped Cream

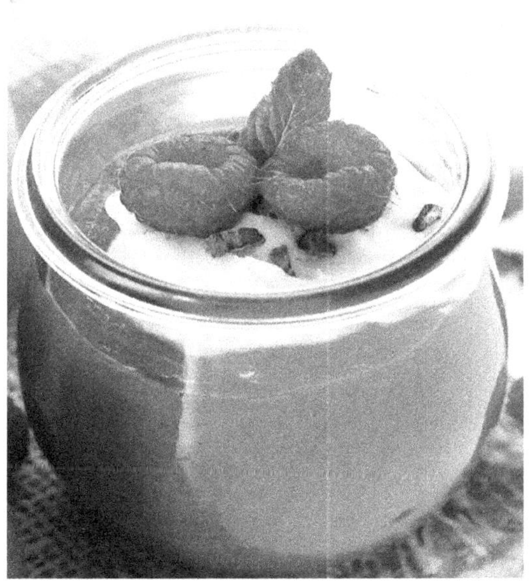

Ingredients:
- 1/2 cup chia seeds

- 1 cup coconut milk
- 1/4 cup unsweetened cocoa powder
- 2 tablespoons maple syrup
- 1/4 teaspoon salt
- 1/2 cup coconut cream
- 1 tablespoon unsweetened shredded coconut

Instructions:
1. In a bowl, mix together chia seeds, coconut milk, cocoa powder, maple syrup, and salt. Refrigerate for 2 hours or overnight.
2. In a separate bowl, whip the coconut cream until smooth and creamy.
3. Top the chia pudding with coconut whipped cream and unsweetened shredded coconut.
4. Enjoy your delicious and healthy vegan chocolate chia pudding.

Low Carb And Keto Friendly Recipes

1. Keto Creamy Chicken And Mushroom Soup

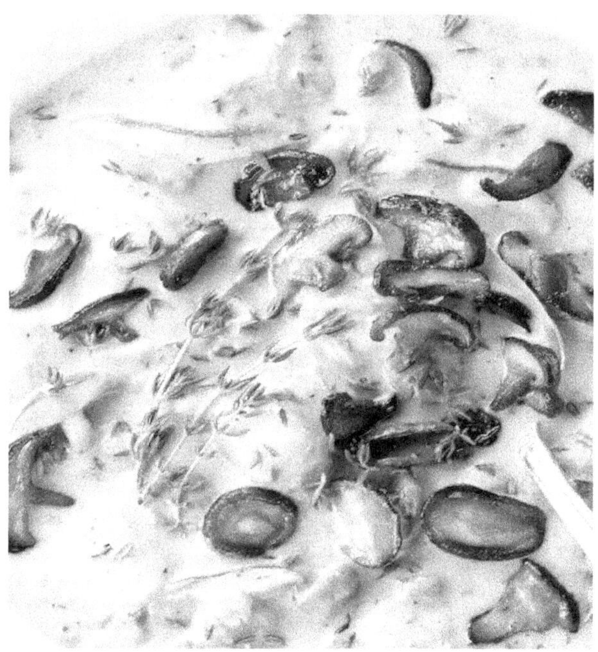

Ingredients:

1 pound boneless, skinless chicken breast or thighs
- 2 cups mixed mushrooms (button, cremini, shiitake)
- 2 tablespoons butter or keto-friendly oil
- 1 onion, diced

- 2 cloves garlic, minced
- 1 cup chicken broth
- 1/2 cup heavy cream or keto-friendly alternative
- 1 teaspoon dried thyme
- Salt and pepper, to taste

Instructions:
1. In a large pot, sauté the chicken, mushrooms, onion, and garlic in butter or oil until the chicken is cooked through and the mushrooms are tender.
2. Add the chicken broth, heavy cream, and thyme. Bring to a simmer and cook for 5-7 minutes or until the soup has thickened slightly.
3. Season with salt and pepper to taste.
4. Serve hot and enjoy!

This recipe is not only delicious, but it's also packed with nutrients and fits perfectly within a PCOS diet. The chicken and mushrooms provide a boost of protein and healthy fats, while the heavy cream adds a rich and creamy texture without the added carbs.

2. Low-Carb Cauliflower Fried Rice With Shrimp

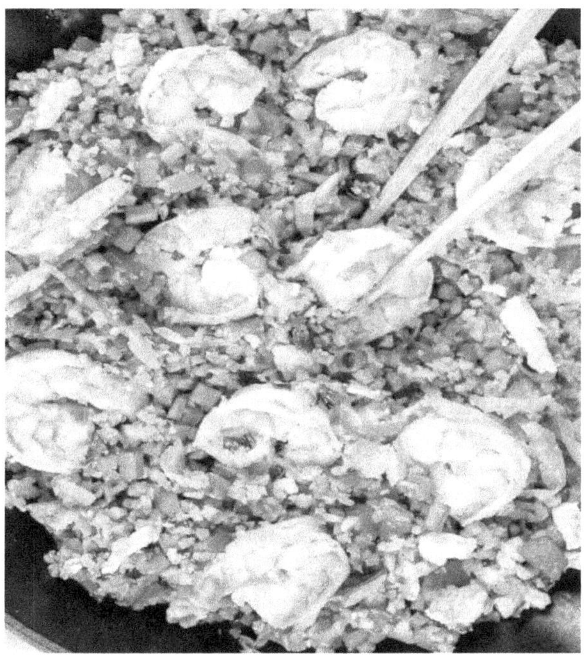

Ingredients:
- 1 head of cauliflower
- 1 cup cooked shrimp
- 2 tablespoons coconut oil
- 1 onion, diced
- 2 cloves garlic, minced
- 1 cup mixed veggies (e.g., peas, carrots, green onions)
- 2 teaspoons soy sauce (make sure it's sugar-free)
- 1 teaspoon sesame oil
- Salt and pepper, to taste

Instructions:

1. Pulse the cauliflower in a food processor until it resembles rice.
2. In a large skillet, heat the coconut oil and sauté the onion, garlic, and mixed veggies until tender.
3. Add the cooked shrimp, cauliflower "rice," soy sauce, and sesame oil. Stir-fry everything together.
4. Season with salt and pepper to taste.
5. Serve hot and enjoy!

This recipe is a game-changer for low-carb and keto-friendly meals. The cauliflower "rice" is a genius substitute for traditional rice, and the shrimp adds a boost of protein.

3. Keto Zucchini Boats With Meatballs And Marinara Sauce

Ingredients:
- 4 zucchinis
- 1 pound meatballs (made with almond flour and Parmesan cheese)
- 1 cup marinara sauce (make sure it's sugar-free)
- 1 cup melted mozzarella cheese (or keto-friendly alternative)
- 1/4 cup chopped fresh parsley
- Salt and pepper, to taste

Instructions:
1. Preheat the oven to 400°F (200°C).

2. Scoop out the zucchinis and fill with meatballs.
3. Pour marinara sauce over the meatballs and top with mozzarella cheese.
4. Bake for 25-30 minutes or until the cheese is melted and bubbly.
5. Sprinkle with parsley and serve hot!

This recipe is a flavorful and satisfying option for a PCOS diet. The zucchinis provide a low-carb and nutritious base, while the meatballs and marinara sauce add a boost of protein and flavor.

4. Low-Carb Spinach And Feta Stuffed Chicken Breast

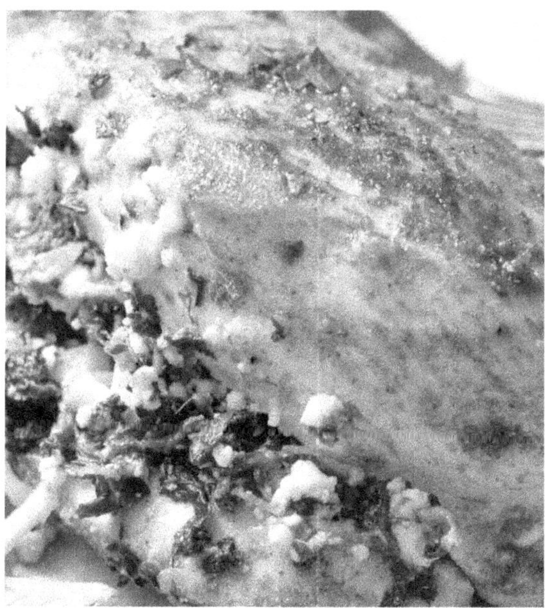

Ingredients:
- 4 boneless, skinless chicken breasts
- 1 package frozen chopped spinach, thawed and drained
- 1/2 cup crumbled feta cheese
- 1/4 cup chopped fresh parsley
- 2 cloves garlic, minced
- 1/2 teaspoon salt
- 1/4 teaspoon black pepper

Instructions:
1. Preheat the oven to 375°F (190°C).
2. In a bowl, mix together spinach, feta cheese, parsley, garlic, salt, and pepper.
3. Stuff each chicken breast with the spinach mixture and bake for 25-30 minutes or until cooked through.

This recipe is a great source of protein, healthy fats, and low-carb veggies, making it an excellent option for a PCOS diet. The spinach and parsley add a boost of antioxidants and fiber, while the feta cheese provides a tangy and creamy flavor.

5. Keto Chocolate Mousse With Coconut Whipped Cream

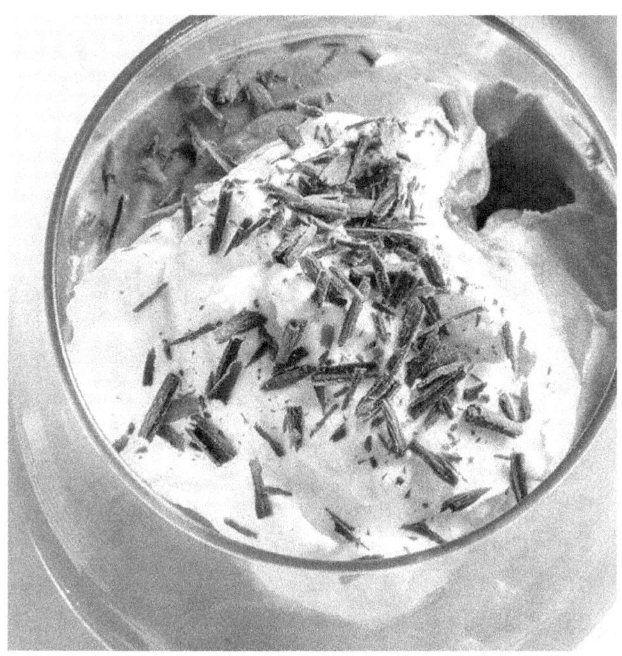

Ingredients:
- 8 ounces dark chocolate (at least 85% cocoa)
- 1/2 cup heavy cream or keto-friendly alternative
- 1/4 cup granulated sweetener (like Swerve or Erythritol)
- 2 large egg whites
- 1/2 cup coconut cream, chilled
- 1 teaspoon vanilla extract

Instructions:
1. In a double boiler, melt the chocolate and sweetener.

2. In a separate bowl, whip the egg whites until stiff peaks form.
3. Fold the egg whites into the chocolate mixture.
4. In a separate bowl, whip the coconut cream until stiff peaks form.
5. Add vanilla extract and mix well.
6. Serve the chocolate mousse with coconut whipped cream.

6. Low-Carb Keto Crab Cakes With Remoulade Sauce

Ingredients:
- 1 pound jumbo lump crab meat
- 1/4 cup almond flour
- 1/4 cup coconut flour
- 1/4 cup granulated sweetener (like Swerve or Erythritol)
- 2 tablespoons mayonnaise
- 1 tablespoon Dijon mustard
- 1 teaspoon Worcestershire sauce
- 1/2 teaspoon Old Bay seasoning
- 1/4 teaspoon salt
- 1/4 teaspoon black pepper
- 2 tablespoons coconut oil
- Remoulade Sauce (made with mayonnaise, ketchup, and herbs)

Instructions:
1. In a bowl, mix together crab meat, almond flour, coconut flour, sweetener, mayonnaise, Dijon

mustard, Worcestershire sauce, Old Bay
seasoning, salt, and pepper.
2. Form into patties and fry in coconut oil until
golden brown.
3. Serve with Remoulade Sauce.

This recipe is a low-carb and keto-friendly twist on
traditional crab cakes. The almond flour and
coconut flour provide a nutritious and low-carb
base, while the crab meat adds a boost of protein
and flavor.

7. Keto Creamy Asparagus And Ham Soup

Ingredients:
- 1 pound fresh asparagus, trimmed
- 1 cup diced ham
- 2 tablespoons butter or keto-friendly oil
- 1 onion, diced
- 2 cloves garlic, minced
- 1 cup chicken broth
- 1/2 cup heavy cream or keto-friendly alternative
- Salt and pepper, to taste

Instructions:
1. In a pot, sauté the asparagus, ham, onion, and
garlic in butter or oil until tender.
2. Add the chicken broth and bring to a boil.
3. Reduce heat and simmer until the asparagus is
tender.

4. Blend the mixture until smooth.
5. Stir in the heavy cream or alternative and season with salt and pepper.

8. Low-Carb Keto Chicken And Vegetable Kabobs With Pesto Sauce

Ingredients:
- 1 pound boneless, skinless chicken breast or thighs
- 1 cup mixed vegetables (bell peppers, zucchini, onions, mushrooms)
- 1/4 cup pesto sauce (made with basil, garlic, and olive oil)
- 2 tablespoons olive oil
- Salt and pepper, to taste

Instructions:
1. Preheat the grill or grill pan to medium-high heat.
2. Thread the chicken and vegetables onto skewers.
3. Brush with olive oil and season with salt and pepper.
4. Grill for 10-12 minutes or until the chicken is cooked through.
5. Serve with pesto sauce.

9. Keto Lemon Bars With A Shortbread Crust

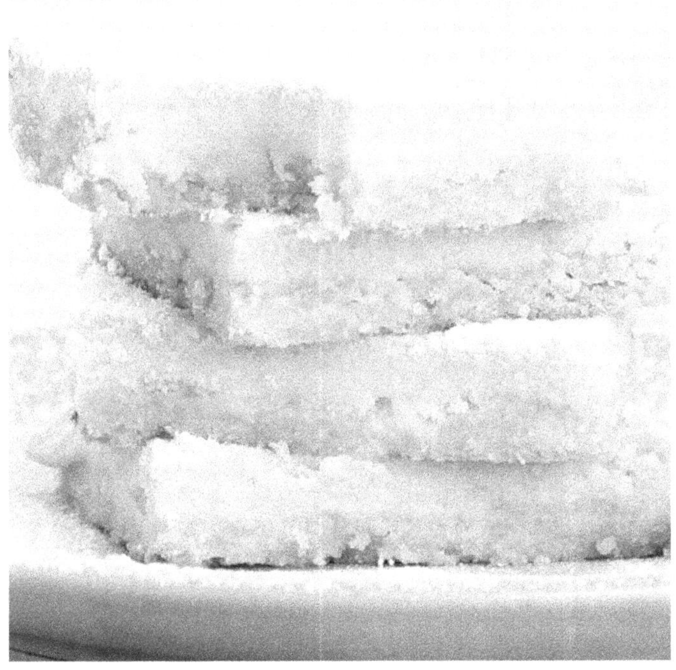

Ingredients:
- 1 1/2 cups almond flour
- 1/4 cup granulated sweetener (like Swerve or Erythritol)
- 1/4 cup unsalted butter, melted
- 2 large eggs
- 1 teaspoon lemon zest
- 2 tablespoons freshly squeezed lemon juice

Instructions:
1. Preheat the oven to 350°F (180°C).

2. Mix the almond flour, sweetener, and melted butter to make the shortbread crust.
3. Press the mixture into a baking dish.
4. Mix the eggs, lemon zest, and lemon juice to make the lemon filling.
5. Pour the filling over the crust.
6. Bake for 20-25 minutes or until the filling is set.

10. Low-Carb Keto Breakfast Skillet With Scrambled Eggs And Avocado

Ingredients:
- 4 eggs
- 1/2 avocado, diced
- 1/2 cup spinach, chopped
- 1/2 cup cherry tomatoes, halved
- 1/4 cup sliced red onion
- 2 slices of bacon, cooked and crumbled
- Salt and pepper, to taste

Instructions:
1. In a skillet, scramble the eggs and set aside.
2. Add the avocado, spinach, cherry tomatoes, and red onion to the skillet.
3. Cook until the vegetables are tender.
4. Add the scrambled eggs and bacon to the skillet.
5. Stir everything together and serve hot.

Chapter Six

Managing Food Cravings And Emotional Eating

These are tips for managing food cravings and emotional eating:

1. Stay hydrated: Sometimes thirst can be mistaken for hunger or cravings. Drink water throughout the day to stay hydrated and reduce cravings.

2. Eat regular meals: Skipping meals can lead to overeating or making unhealthy choices later in the day. Eat balanced meals and snacks to keep your hunger and cravings under control.

3. Identify triggers: Pay attention to when and why you experience cravings or emotional eating. Is it when you're stressed? Bored? Around certain people or in certain situations? Once you identify your triggers, you can develop strategies to manage them.

4. Find healthy alternatives: If you're craving something specific like ice cream or chips, find a healthier alternative like Greek yogurt or air-popped popcorn.

5. Practice mindful eating: Pay attention to your hunger and fullness cues, savor your food, and eat slowly. This can help you enjoy your food more and feel more satisfied.

6. Get enough sleep: Lack of sleep can increase cravings for unhealthy foods. Aim for 7-8 hours of sleep per night to help regulate your appetite and metabolism.

7. Get support: Share your struggles with a friend or family member and ask for their support. Having someone to hold you accountable and provide encouragement can make a big difference.

8. Keep healthy snacks on hand: Prepare healthy snacks like fruits, nuts, and veggies with hummus to curb cravings and prevent unhealthy choices.

9. Find healthy coping mechanisms: Instead of turning to food when you're stressed or emotional, try going for a walk, practicing yoga, or engaging in a hobby you enjoy.

10. Be kind to yourself: Remember that it's okay to indulge sometimes. Don't beat yourself up over a slip-up - just get back on track and keep moving forward.

By incorporating these tips,women can learn how to manage food cravings and emotional eating, develop healthier relationships with food, and achieve their health and wellness goals.

Lifestyle And Self-care

Lifestyle:
1. Regular exercise: Aim for at least 30 minutes of moderate-intensity exercise per day to improve insulin sensitivity and hormone balance.

2. Stress management: Engage in stress-reducing activities like yoga, meditation, or deep breathing exercises.

3. Sleep: Aim for 7-8 hours of sleep per night to regulate hormones and metabolism.

4. Limit alcohol and caffeine: Excessive consumption can worsen PCOS symptoms.

Self-care:
1. Prioritize mental health: Seek support from a therapist or counselor to address emotional struggles.

2. Practice self-compassion: Treat yourself with kindness and understanding, just as you would a close friend.
3. Engage in activities you enjoy: Make time for hobbies, passions, and creative pursuits.

4. Set boundaries: Learn to say "no" and prioritize your own needs and well-being.

Stress Management Techniques

1. Deep Breathing Exercises: Take slow, deliberate breaths in through your nose and out through your mouth, focusing on the sensation of the breath.

2. Progressive Muscle Relaxation: Tense and then relax different muscle groups in your body, starting with your toes and moving up to your head.

3. Mindfulness Meditation: Focus your attention on the present moment, without judgment, and let go of worries about the past or future.

4. Yoga: Practice physical postures, breathing techniques, and meditation to reduce stress and improve overall well-being.

5. Journaling: Write down your thoughts and feelings to process and release them.

6. Grounding Techniques: Use your senses to ground yourself in the present moment, such as focusing on the feeling of your feet on the ground or the sounds around you.

7. Exercise: Engage in physical activity to reduce stress and improve mood.

8. Seek Social Support: Connect with friends, family, or a therapist for emotional support.

9. Time Management: Prioritize tasks, set boundaries, and take breaks to manage stress.

10. Self-Care: Make time for activities that bring you joy and relaxation, such as reading, taking a bath, or listening to music.

Remember, everyone is unique, and what works for one person may not work for another. Experiment with different techniques to find what works best for you.

Regular Exercise And Physical Activities For PCOS Management

1. Aerobic Exercise: Activities like brisk walking, cycling, swimming, and dancing can improve insulin sensitivity and cardiovascular health.

2. Resistance Training: Weightlifting, bodyweight exercises, or resistance band exercises can help build muscle and improve insulin sensitivity.

3. High-Intensity Interval Training (HIIT): Short bursts of intense exercise followed by brief rest periods can improve insulin sensitivity and weight management.

4. Yoga: Combines physical postures, breathing techniques, and meditation to reduce stress, improve flexibility, and regulate hormones.

5. Pilates: Focuses on core strength, flexibility, and body control to improve posture, balance, and overall physical fitness.

6. Brisk Walking: Regular brisk walking can improve insulin sensitivity, weight management, and cardiovascular health.

7. Swimming: Low-impact exercise that improves cardiovascular health, insulin sensitivity, and weight management.

8. Cycling: Indoor or outdoor cycling can improve cardiovascular health, insulin sensitivity, and weight management.

9. Dance-Based Workouts: Fun and energetic workouts like Zumba or Hip Hop Abs can improve cardiovascular health, insulin sensitivity, and weight management.

10. Strength Training: Building muscle mass through strength training can improve insulin sensitivity and overall health.

Remember to consult a healthcare provider before starting any new exercise program, especially if you have any underlying health conditions. Aim for at least 150 minutes of moderate-intensity exercise or 75 minutes of vigorous-intensity exercise per week.

Chapter Seven

Sleep And Relaxation Strategies

Sleep Strategies:
1. Establish a consistent sleep schedule
2. Create a bedtime routine to signal the body for sleep
3. Optimize the sleep environment (cool, dark, quiet)
4. Avoid screens and electronic devices before bedtime
5. Limit caffeine and alcohol intake
6. Try relaxation techniques, such as deep breathing or progressive muscle relaxation, before bed
7. Consider keeping a sleep diary to track patterns and identify areas for improvement

Relaxation Strategies:
1. Deep Breathing Exercises: Focus on slow, deliberate breaths to calm the mind and body

2. Progressive Muscle Relaxation: Tense and release each muscle group to release physical tension

3. Mindfulness Meditation: Focus on the present moment, without judgment, to reduce stress and anxiety

4. Yoga: Combine physical postures, breathing techniques, and meditation to promote relaxation and reduce stress

5. Visualization: Imagine a peaceful, relaxing scene to distract from stressful thoughts and promote relaxation

6. Listening to Calming Music or Nature Sounds: Soothe the mind and body with calming audio

7. Aromatherapy: Inhale essential oils like lavender or chamomile to promote relaxation

8. Body Scan: Lie down and focus on each body part, starting from toes and moving up to head, letting go of any tension

9. Hot Bath or Shower: Soak in warm water or take a relaxing shower to unwind and relax muscles **Read stories:** Escape into a good story or informative content to distract from stressful thoughts.

Mindful Eating And Self-Care Practices

Mindful Eating Practices:
1. Eat slowly and savor your food
2. Pay attention to hunger and fullness cues
3. Eliminate distractions while eating (TV, phone, etc.)
4. Choose nutrient-dense foods
5. Practice gratitude for your food and body
6. Recognize emotional eating triggers and develop healthier coping mechanisms
7. Stay hydrated throughout the day
8. Limit processed and high-sugar foods
9. Cook at home using whole ingredients
10. Enjoy your favorite foods in moderation

Self-Care Practices:
1. Prioritize sleep and aim for 7-8 hours per night
2. Engage in physical activity that brings you joy (walking, yoga, dancing, etc.)
3. Schedule time for relaxation and stress reduction (meditation, deep breathing, etc.)
4. Connect with nature and spend time outdoors
5. Practice self-compassion and challenge negative self-talk
6. Set boundaries and prioritize your own needs
7. Engage in creative activities (art, writing, music, etc.)
8. Take breaks and practice self-care throughout the day

9. Seek support from loved ones, therapy, or support groups
10. Celebrate your accomplishments and acknowledge your strengths

Remember, mindful eating and self-care are journeys, and it's essential to be patient and kind to yourself. Start with small changes and gradually work your way towards a more balanced and nourishing relationship with food and your body.

Cooking Guides And Methods

Cooking Methods
- Grilling: Preheat grill to medium-high heat. Cook for 5-7 minutes per side, or until cooked through.
- Roasting: Preheat the oven to 400°F (200°C). Cook for 20-25 minutes, or until tender and golden brown.
- Sautéing: Heat oil in a pan over medium-high heat. Cook for 3-5 minutes, or until tender and lightly browned.
- Steaming: Bring water to a boil. Reduce heat and steam for 5-7 minutes, or until tender.

Cooking Times
- Vegetables:
    - Leafy greens: 2-3 minutes
    - Broccoli: 3-5 minutes
    - Bell peppers: 5-7 minutes
- Proteins:
    - Chicken breast: 5-7 minutes

  - Salmon filet: 4-6 minutes
  - Tofu: 3-5 minutes

Meal Prep Tips
- Chop vegetables and proteins in advance
- Cook grains and beans in bulk
- Portion meals into individual containers
- Label and date containers for easy storage

Kitchen Essentials
- Good quality pots and pans
- Sharp knives and cutting boards
- Measuring cups and spoons
- Spices and herbs (e.g. turmeric, cumin, basil)

Conclusion

Living with PCOS can be challenging, but it's not impossible to manage. By making simple changes to your diet and lifestyle, you can take control of your symptoms and improve your overall health. The PCOS Diet Cookbook for Women is designed to help you do just that.

Throughout this book, we've explored the importance of nutrition in managing PCOS. We've discussed how a balanced diet can help regulate blood sugar, insulin, and hormones, reducing symptoms like weight gain, acne, and irregular periods. We've also shared delicious and easy-to-make recipes that incorporate whole foods, healthy fats, and protein sources.

But the PCOS Diet Cookbook for Women is more than just a collection of recipes. It's a comprehensive guide to managing PCOS through diet and lifestyle changes. We've covered topics like mindful eating, self-care, and stress management, all of which are essential for overall health and well-being.

By following the principles outlined in this book, you can:

- Regulate your blood sugar and insulin levels
- Reduce androgen hormones and alleviate symptoms like acne and excess hair growth

- Improve your menstrual cycle and fertility
- Boost your mood and energy levels
- Support your overall health and well-being

Remember, managing PCOS is a journey, and it's okay to take it one step at a time. Start by making small changes to your diet and lifestyle, and gradually work your way towards a healthier, happier you.

Don't be afraid to seek support from loved ones, healthcare professionals, or online communities. Connect with other women who understand what you're going through, and learn from their experiences.

Most importantly, be kind to yourself. Living with PCOS can be challenging, but it doesn't define your worth or identity. You are strong, capable, and deserving of love, care, and respect – from yourself and others.

In conclusion, the PCOS Diet Cookbook for Women is a tool to help you take control of your health and well-being. It's a reminder that you have the power to make positive changes in your life, one meal at a time. So go ahead, take the first step, and start cooking your way to a healthier, happier you.

Appendix

7-Days Meal Plan

Day 1:
- Breakfast: Overnight oats with berries and walnuts
- Lunch: Grilled chicken salad with mixed greens, veggies, and avocado
- Dinner: Baked salmon with sweet potato and green beans

Day 2:
- Breakfast: Scrambled eggs with spinach and whole wheat toast
- Lunch: Lentil soup with whole grain bread and a side salad
- Dinner: Grilled turkey burger on a whole grain bun with roasted veggies

Day 3:
- Breakfast: Greek yogurt with berries and granola
- Lunch: Grilled chicken wrap with mixed greens and whole wheat wrap
- Dinner: Slow cooker chili with quinoa and mixed veggies

Day 4:
- Breakfast: Smoothie bowl with protein powder, almond milk, and mixed berries
- Lunch: Turkey and avocado wrap with mixed greens and whole wheat wrap

- Dinner: Grilled shrimp with brown rice and
steamed broccoli

Day 5:
- Breakfast: Avocado toast with scrambled eggs
and cherry tomatoes
- Lunch: Grilled chicken salad with mixed greens,
veggies, and whole grain crackers
- Dinner: Baked chicken thighs with roasted
Brussels sprouts and sweet potatoes

Day 6:
- Breakfast: Omelette with mushrooms, spinach,
and whole wheat toast
- Lunch: Lentil and veggie curry with brown rice and
whole grain naan
- Dinner: Grilled salmon with roasted asparagus
and quinoa

Day 7:
- Breakfast: Breakfast burrito with scrambled eggs,
black beans, and avocado
- Lunch: Grilled chicken and quinoa bowl with
roasted veggies and mixed greens
- Dinner: Baked cod with roasted bell peppers and
brown rice

Grocery Lists And Pantry Staples

Grocery List:

- **Fresh produce:**
    - Leafy greens (spinach, kale, collard greens)
    - Berries (blueberries, strawberries, raspberries)
    - Citrus fruits (oranges, grapefruits, lemons)
    - Cruciferous vegetables (broccoli, cauliflower, cauliflower)
- Proteins:
    - Grass-fed beef
    - Wild-caught salmon
    - Organic chicken
    - Tofu

- **Whole grains:**
    - Brown rice
    - Quinoa
    - Whole wheat bread
    - Whole grain pasta

- **Healthy fats:**
    - Avocados
    - Nuts and seeds (almonds, chia seeds, flax seeds)
    - Olive oil

- **Dairy:**
    - Greek yogurt
    - Cottage cheese
- Pantry staples:
    - Canned beans (black beans, chickpeas, lentils)
    - Canned tomatoes
    - Coconut oil
    - Spices and herbs (turmeric, cinnamon, basil)

Pantry Staples:
- Grains:
- Brown rice
- Quinoa
- Whole wheat pasta
- Oats

- Canned goods:
- Black beans
- Chickpeas
- Lentils
- Diced tomatoes

- Nuts and seeds:
- Almonds
- Chia seeds
- Flax seeds
- Walnuts
- Baking supplies:
  - Almond flour
  - Coconut flour
  - Oat flour

- Snacks:
- Nut butters (peanut butter, almond butter)
- Dried fruits (dates, apricots, prunes)
- Energy balls (made with oats, nuts, and seeds)

Conversion Chart

Measurement Conversions

- 1 cup = 8 ounces = 250ml
- 1/2 cup = 4 ounces = 125ml
- 1/4 cup = 2 ounces = 60ml
- 1 tablespoon (tbsp) = 3 teaspoons (tsp) = 15ml
- 1 teaspoon (tsp) = 5ml

Weight Conversions

- 1 pound (lb) = 16 ounces (oz) = 450g
- 1 ounce (oz) = 28g

Temperature Conversions

- Fahrenheit (°F) to Celsius (°C):
    - 200°F = 90°C
    - 180°F = 80°C
    - 350°F = 175°C
- Celsius (°C) to Fahrenheit (°F):
    - 20°C = 68°F
    - 25°C = 77°F
    - 30°C = 86°F

Volume Conversions

- 1 quart (qt) = 4 cups = 1 liter (L)
- 1 pint (pt) = 2 cups = 0.5L
- 1 cup = 8 fluid ounces (fl oz) = 0.25L

Meal Plan Template

Monday:
- Breakfast:

____

____

- Lunch:

____

____

- Dinner:

____

____

- Snacks:

____

____

Tuesday:
- Breakfast:

____

____

- Lunch:

____

____

- Dinner:

____

____

- Snacks:

____

____

Wednesday:
- Breakfast:

____

____

- Lunch:

____

____

- Dinner:

____

- Snacks:

____

Thursday:
- Breakfast:

____

- Lunch:

____

- Dinner:

____

- Snacks:

____

Friday:
- Breakfast:

____

- Lunch:

____

- Dinner:

____

- Snacks:

____

____

Saturday:
- Breakfast:

____

____

- Lunch:

____

____

- Dinner:

____

____

- Snacks:

____

____

Sunday:
- Breakfast:

____

____

- Lunch:

____

____

- Dinner:

____

____

- Snacks:

____

____